I08791133

Studies in Rhetorics and Feminisms

Series Editors, Cheryl Glenn and Shirley Wilson Logan

WRiTING CHiLDBiRTH

Women's Rhetorical Agency in Labor and Online

KIM HENSLEY OWENS

Southern Illinois University Press
Carbondale

Printed in the United States of America

18 17 16 15 4 3 2 1

Cover illustration: *Le ciel à la terre* (Heaven to Earth), oil monoprint, by Kay M. Pick (Zivkovich), © 2014

Library of Congress Cataloging-in-Publication Data

Owens, Kim Hensley, 1974–
Writing childbirth : women's rhetorical agency in labor and online / Kim Hensley Owens.
pages cm. — (Studies in rhetorics and feminisms)
Includes bibliographical references and index.
ISBN 978-0-8093-3405-6 (paperback)
ISBN 0-8093-3405-4 (paperback)
ISBN 978-0-8093-3406-3 (ebook)
1. Childbirth—United States—Psychological aspects. 2. Childbirth—United States—Computer network resources. 3. Patients' writings—United States—History and criticism. 4. Birth plans—United States. 5. Rhetoric—United States. 6. Internet in medicine—United States. 7. Communication in medicine—United States. 8. Communication in obstetrics—United States. I. Title.
RG652.O94 2015
618.2—dc23 2014043790

The paper used in this publication meets the minimum requirements of American National Standard for Information Sciences—Permanence of Paper for Printed Library Materials, ANSI Z39.48-1992. ♾

For Luke, Ethan, and Eleni,
who make my world spin

CONTENTS

PREFACE

I was almost born in a Volkswagen bus. My parents were camping an hour from the nearest hospital, two from "their" hospital and home. My mother, nine months pregnant, awoke to pangs. She told my father she thought she was in labor, but he said, "No, it's just heartburn from the chili dogs." Within the hour she was shaking him awake again, insisting that the pangs were labor, that she knew she was in labor. Realization dawning, my father helped my mother into the VW and sped toward town. Contractions three minutes apart, they raced past hospital number one, deciding they had more time. Contractions two minutes apart, they veered into the waiting room at St. Joseph's Hospital in Tucson, Arizona. I was born shortly thereafter, my mother giving birth with no more assistance than a small cut by a Dr. William Oats and my father's encouraging grin.

I share my mother's story because it represents, for me, an important moment of feminist rhetorical agency. Readers may notice that my mother asserted her rhetorical agency twice before anyone (even she) fully believed or acted upon the message that she was in labor—that her own embodied experience was the authoritative interpretation of the situation. With that element highlighted, this story could be framed to exemplify the trope of "female" intuitive, bodily knowing versus "male" dismissal of such knowledge. The story can also be framed differently, however, and read as a tale of danger thwarted by the nick-of-time hospital arrival; as anecdotal proof of women's ability to labor naturally; as an indication that women need both medical assistance and partner support in birth; as a testament to labor's unpredictable schedule; or as a demonstration of experience being (re)constructed through narrative. While my mother's story differs from my own experiences and from those of the women whose writing I examine throughout this book, I hear echoes of those stories in this one, hints of many of the themes and rhetorical positions in modern American childbirth and childbirth writing.

As a feminist rhetorician, I take seriously the obligation to provide context for readers about my own position and experience. By sharing this story, I begin to acknowledge my positioning in a book that explores how scholars, authors, and especially everyday women write about and assert their rhetorical agency in relation to childbirth. The book is not about me or my experiences, but because my experiences with childbirth—including my awareness of this story—affect my perceptions of the material and rhetorical aspects of childbirth and of women's agency and inevitably inflect the project as a whole, I make my experiences and perspective as transparent as possible. In the epilogue, I share my own birth stories, refracted through the arguments made and lessons learned through the research for this project. These stories illustrate, in context, various rhetorical features and functions of modern American birth culture and women's birth stories.

Stories provide ways for people to frame and understand their lives; they help people place themselves and others in relation to one another and to their cultures. Childbirth stories include not only those stories women share about their birth experiences but also the stories medicine tells about childbirth, the stories various cultural texts tell about childbirth, and the stories women tell themselves and others about their hopes and expectations for birth. Women absorb, respond to, and share many kinds of childbirth stories, with a variety of rhetorical and material effects that extend far beyond childbirth itself. Understanding these stories and their influences helps us better understand women's roles in society, the cultural scripts surrounding those roles, and women's ways of asserting feminist rhetorical agency within and against those cultural scripts.

This book grew out of my need to make sense of theory, to make the theoretical speak to the concrete, and vice versa, and it evolved into an opportunity to examine childbirth as a rhetorical exigence and to bring women's agency and childbirth into broader discussions of rhetoric, feminism, and health. The idea sparked as I read Naomi Wolf's *Misconceptions* and Isabel Allende's *Paula* for pleasure while taking an increased scholarly interest in the work of Judith Butler and Joan W. Scott; these disparate works and authors helped shape this book, which is intended to honor women's choices as writers and as birthing women.

A few notes about how I've handled women's voices and identification information in the text: in order to preserve the voices of the women whose online birth narratives, birth plans, and survey responses I cite, I have left their writing intact, including any abbreviations, typos, and spelling errors. However, I have corrected any book titles or authors' names, and where meaning seemed potentially unclear, I have made very small changes or added notes to explain abbreviations. Women I surveyed had the option to use their real names or pseudonyms of their choice. For consistency's sake,

I refer to all survey respondents and all narrative authors by first names only, even if they gave consent for their last names to be included. In some instances, online birth narratives do not include even a mother's first name but do provide the child's name. In these cases, I refer to the woman as "[child's name]'s mother."

Some of the work in the following chapters has been previously published. A version of chapter 3 was published as "Confronting Rhetorical Disability: A Critical Analysis of Five Women's Birth Plans" in *Written Communication* 26.3 (2009): 247–72 (originally published online 22 December 2008, at doi:10.1177/0741088308329217; now available at http://wcx.sagepub.com/content/26/3/247). In addition, portions of material that has now been developed into chapters 4 and 5 appeared as a chapter called "Revelations and Representations: Birth Stories and Motherhood on the Internet" in *Textual Mothers/Maternal Texts: Mothering in Contemporary Women's Literatures*, ed. Elizabeth Podnieks and Andrea O'Reilly (West Waterloo, ON: Wilfrid Laurier University Press, 2010), 349–64 (http://www.wlupress.wlu.ca/press/Catalog/podnieks.shtml), used with permission.

A final note: books often rely upon pregnancy and childbirth metaphors to describe the process of projects being conceived, carried to term, and brought into the world. For a project in which writing about pregnancy and childbirth figure prominently, this metaphor might even be expected. But after studying and writing about childbirth and childbirth writing and experiencing pregnancy and childbirth twice in the midst of that process, I find the metaphor inadequate. The process of writing and researching this book has taken significantly more time and has been more intellectually, emotionally, and even physically challenging than bearing either of my children. On the other end of that comparison spectrum, while I celebrate coming to the end of this long process and look forward to seeing what life this book will lead, that feeling cannot compare to the sense of wonder and anticipation I feel watching my children's lives unfold.

ACKNOWLEDGMENTS

I am indebted to many incredibly generous and intelligent readers, several of whom read multiple iterations of this book over the years. Any errors, omissions, or inelegant prose in this text are my sole responsibility, but any insightful arguments or elegant turns of phrase are no doubt influenced by the comments of those friends and colleagues who have contributed their time and expertise to making this a better book. This project has spanned several years—more than one writing group, more than one kind of support.

Thank you:

To my mom and dad, for a great birth story and everything else.

To Derek Van Ittersum, who picked me up when this project fell down and who has made the mud puddles of everyone's revisions into fun intellectual stomping grounds with our writing group, the Flying Geckos. To the other geckos: Kory Ching, Lauren Marshall Bowen, and Peter Mortensen (and, for a time, Chad Wickman). To Skype, Google Drive, and Gmail, for keeping these brilliant people's words in my inbox and their voices, laughter, and ideas in my ears. Your support has been immeasurably important.

To Amy Hamilton, my *comadre*, for years and years of being there and being awesome.

To Christa Olson, Amy Wan, and Janine Solberg, for virtual support on everything.

To Jamie White-Farnham, Cathryn Molloy, and Tim Amidon, beloved students in my rhetorics of/and reproduction graduate seminar, for getting it.

To Debbie Hawhee and Peter Mortensen, who together and separately gave acres of time as well as rich, challenging feedback to the first iteration of this project. To my dear friends Janine Solberg and Amy Wan, again, without whom there would never have been a first draft, and to other PDawG members: Elizabeth Baldridge, John Hudson, Lance Massey, Jim Purdy. To other early readers: Gail Hawisher, Cathy Prendergast, and Leslie Reagan.

To my colleagues at the University of Rhode Island: Bob Schwegler, whose good cheer brightens even the dimmest of hallways; Jeremiah Dyehouse; Nedra Reynolds; Caroline Gottschalk Druschke; Michael Pennell (even though he left); Libby Miles; Heather Johnson; Helen O'Grady; and Jean Zipke. Their support of all aspects of my/our work is unparalleled.

To my poli-sci pals, for listening and lunches and laughs: Brian Krueger, Marc Hutchison, and Kristin Johnson.

To URI, for time: specifically, three semesters of reduced teaching in my pretenure years. To URI's Council for Research Career Enhancement Grant, which provided support for work on this project.

To Donna Hayden, Lauri Hayden, and Teresa Bertram, who each set the bar for administrative assistance extremely, extremely high.

To editors Shirley Wilson Logan, Cheryl Glenn, Kristine Priddy, and the outside reviewer whose feedback helped me refine this project.

To the wonderful book shepherds at Southern Illinois University Press, who found the right cover image and helped me every step of the way.

To Julie Bush, for incredible attention to detail at the copyediting stage.

To my midwives. To Kate Scott. To all the women who wrote online birth narratives and completed my survey.

To Judith Brysk, for permission to use information from my 2005 interview with her about birth plans.

To the teachers who keep my children delighted about their worlds while I am at work.

And finally, to my little family: Ethan, whose elaborate visions and passion for creation I could never have predicted; Eleni, my red-headed sprite of a daughter, whose love of life is infectious and insanely loud; Ascha the cat, who alone among our cats kept me company as I wrote; and Luke, who performs breakfast miracles before my brain even turns on each day, who acts as my personal librarian on top of his real job, and who makes everything in our lives, from the dryer to dinner to my sentences, better. Thank you for all of the everything.

Writing Childbirth

INTRODUCTiON

Writing Birth—Asserting Rhetorical Agency

The rhetoric of childbirth is multivalenced, is infused with dominant discourses, and illustrates how women's rhetorical agency works beyond occupying preexisting subject positions. As women write their way into childbirth—into understanding themselves as birthing women and mothers within a culture—they sometimes occupy conflicting or shifting positions.

In the pages that follow, I examine women's ways of writing childbirth—their attempts to make their voices heard and to assert their rhetorical agency before, during, and after childbirth—and the ways their rhetorical and material choices interact with one another and with dominant norms and discourses of childbirth. I argue that the rhetorical space of the hospital, in concert with dominant discourses and the hegemonic nature of Western medicine in the United States, obstructs individual women's abilities to successfully assert agency-as-power in the moments of childbirth. Women, however, continue to write—ever more, and online, for wider audiences than ever before—about their experiences with childbirth.

Although childbirth is an ideologically significant experience across all cultures, and although modern American women increasingly write about childbirth (in birth plans and online birth narratives, for example), both childbirth itself and women's writings about childbirth are undertheorized from a rhetorical perspective. This book offers readers in a variety of fields (for example, rhetoric and composition, women's/gender studies, rhetorics of health and medicine, and nurse-midwifery) a fresh understanding of individual women's agency-making tactics in this area of reproductive health / reproductive choice. These tactics can be understood in Michel de Certeau's terms: birthing women writing about childbirth are "others" who rely on "tactics" as they seek, but do not always achieve, agency over a dominant culture (for example, hospital birth), while the dominant culture/hospital constitutes a "scientific institution" that uses broad-ranging "strategies" to assert its power (xix). Individuals' (others') preferences and experiences are not included in the discourse of biomedicine, and the tactics of those who seek to add their preferences or experience to that biomedical hegemony are not always effective, yet these rhetorical efforts are, I argue, meaningful as everyday rhetorical practices and also have potential to effect change over time.

My argument rests on several interlocking contentions about rhetorical agency: (1) women write birth plans in an effort to assert rhetorical agency over their own births, with mixed, usually less-than-successful results; (2) many women who write birth stories and post them online do so in part to retroactively reassert rhetorical agency over their own births, as well as to offer other women ways of understanding, writing their ways into, and asserting feminist rhetorical agency over their own birth experiences; and (3) both kinds of writing are feminist acts. Understanding these writings as both feminist and rhetorical allows scholars to view feminist rhetorical agency as a series of assertions over time and space rather than exclusively as specific instantiations in or for a particular moment or event. Further, I argue that the Internet, or, here, the online spaces that influence or host women's birth writings, help to distribute—in terms of spreading and inspiring, but sometimes also in terms of spreading thin or limiting—feminist rhetorical agency.

Writing Childbirth contributes to understandings of feminist rhetorical agency and understandings of what I call everyday rhetorics of health and medicine. These rhetorics matter personally and politically. Expanding upon Adrienne Rich's claim that childbirth choices and practices are always political, I demonstrate the various political effects of childbirth writing and how these political effects interact with personal effects. To give readers entrée into the political effects of women's birth choices and birth-related writing, I begin with this recent story.

RHETORICAL AGENCY AND INSTITUTIONAL POWER: THE LIGHTS' STORY

On 21 July 2011, a newborn baby in Illinois named Ruth Light was taken from her parents, Ryan and Melissa Light, and placed into foster care by Child Protective Services. The Illinois CPS cited neglect, which it determined after Ruth's hospitalization when she was a few hours old. The Lights had taken their baby to the hospital a few hours after her birth—a home birth—because she seemed to be in pain.

Ruth's shoulder had been injured during birth—she had had an unanticipated childbirth complication known as shoulder dystocia, where a baby's shoulders become lodged behind the mother's pubic bone and require the birth attendant to manually extract the baby. Shoulder dystocia occurs without warning and affects 0.6–1.4 percent of babies with a birth weight between 5 lb., 8 oz., and 8 lb., 13 oz., and 5–9 percent of babies born weighing more (Baxley and Gabbo 1707). Deliveries complicated by shoulder dystocia carry risks of additional injury to the baby. Ruth Light suffered nerve damage, which her parents discovered when they sought treatment the night of her birth.

It is important to point out that neither the shoulder dystocia nor the iatrogenic (caregiver-caused) nerve damage were the result of Ruth's being born at home. Both the complication and its resultant problems occur in hospital births attended by physicians, which represent the vast majority of births (approximately 91 percent of all births) in the United States. As a case in point: the Gaskin Maneuver, one obstetric maneuver employed to successfully handle shoulder dystocia, was developed by Ina May Gaskin, herself a home-birth midwife. CPS does not remove children from their parents' homes when they suffer injuries in hospital births, and they did not take Ruth away because she had a birth injury. Rather, CPS deemed Ruth's parents neglectful because of their choice to birth at home rather than at the culturally dominant location of the hospital. The Lights' act of resistance, of asserting the agency to birth at home, against dominant norms and expectations, led to their daughter's removal from their care.

Ryan and Melissa Light fought the decision on legal, medical, and logical grounds. While visiting their daughter at every available opportunity—mere hours (supervised) a day for months, Melissa set up a Facebook page, "Bring Ruth Home," where she posted this story:

> Aug. 13th—Ruth Abigail Light was born at home on July 21st at 7:38PM. She weighed 7 lbs. 10 oz. and was 20 inches long. During the birth, her shoulders were stuck momentarily (Shoulder Dystocia) but once they were free, she came right out. Ruth was doing well but a few hours later she seemed to be fussier than usual and we decided to take her in to get her checked out just to be sure. We took her to the ER in the middle of the night. Over the next few days, they told us that her arms had nerve damage from her shoulders getting stuck and a couple of days later, someone filed a complaint against us citing medical neglect for having

> her at home vs. the recommended C-section since she was breech. Since that time, Ruth has had every test possible run and so far, she seems to be doing very well. Her arms are recovering and she is a very content baby.
>
> Unfortunately, the State of Illinois took her into custody as a result of the complaint and she has been in foster care for over a week. During that time, we were only allowed to see her twice for a couple of hours. Thankfully, as of Aug. 9th, she was placed with Melissa's parents and we are now allowed to see her for a few hours each day. This has obviously been a very hard situation for our entire family. We ask for your prayers as we walk this road and especially for a full recovery for Ruth. We will keep this site updated with any new information as it develops so that everyone can stay in touch. Thank you to all of you for your endless support.
>
> Ryan, Melissa and Ruth

In taking her story to a publicly accessible Facebook page, Melissa made a Web 2.0 decision that allowed her to assert rhetorical agency over her daughter's birth and story in the face of actions that were far beyond her ability as an individual to counteract. Through the Facebook page, the family gained 2,896 supporters, some of whom wrote letters to the district attorney on their behalf (as I did). Other supporters provided emotionally encouraging messages, asked for updates, and occasionally posted about other home-birth or CPS-related injustices. Eight months after her birth, Ruth was returned to the home in which she had been born.[1]

The Lights' story hints at the various ways women's individual rhetorical agency with regard to health and medicine is complicated or compromised by institutional power and the ideological force of cultural expectations;[2] women are disciplined, in the Foucauldian sense, into particular choices and orientations to childbirth, and resistance can lead to further disciplining. Melissa Light was able to exercise her agency in terms of deciding to birth at home, but when a birth injury occurred, she was punished for that resistance—even though a hospital birth neither prevents nor handles such birth injuries more safely. In Illinois, where home birth is neither legal nor illegal for birthing mothers (although it is illegal for certified professional midwives to attend home births there), and in the United States, where birth choices are delimited by a strong cultural preference for medical assistance (as well as by hospital hierarchies and insurance companies), women's rhetorical agency as birthing mothers is also delimited, circumscribed by cultural forces and cultural scripts that can supersede individual enactments of choice.

CHILDBIRTH: AN EVERYDAY YET EXTRAORDINARY EVENT

> [G]iving birth to Joshua was the most wonderful and memorible[3] experience of my life. (Kim)

> Then came the words that made me burst into tears, c-section. (Sandra)

> The contractions finally came so quick that I couldn't even change my clothes to get to the hospital. I then had the most excrucuciating pain, the top of my stomach got soft; empty feeling. I felt the baby's head and then decided that I was having this baby at home. I sat on the side of the toilet, pushed once then my water broke then another push and caught my baby girl. She didn't cry, just looked around, looked at me and was as if she had this look on her face like finally I get to see you! I wiped her with a towel, wrapped her up, held her against me, and called 911. They showed up, amazed how good she looked, and once I got in the ambulance, she nursed all the way to the hospital. (Jesse)

Childbirth is one of the most extraordinary of ordinary events. It happens more than ten thousand times a day in the United States, more than three hundred thousand times a day across the globe, and yet for each individual, it remains a powerful, life-changing affair. The excerpts above hint at the ways each story is at once unique and profound, as will those shared throughout this book. Although to some extent childbirth is a "natural" phenomenon that should change little over time, rapid changes in technologies, beliefs, and practices have resulted in significant and increasing material changes in American birth over the last century and a half. Among these changes: birth has primarily shifted from the home to the hospital; nearly all hospital labors are monitored with an external fetal monitor; approximately 80 percent of women receive epidural analgesia during labor; and 32 percent of women give birth via cesarean—often in unplanned cesareans, like Sandra's.

As even these brief statistics illustrate, American childbirth is at present deeply entrenched in the discourse of biomedicine, by which I mean not only language but also technologies, interactions, practices, and orientations. This entrenchment has changed childbirth and affects how women write, read, and learn about childbirth. Modern Americans experience dominant discourses of childbirth through popular media, histories, medical and instructional texts, and interactions with care providers, one another, and online. Each of these disparate encounters helps to subtly (and not so subtly) imprint ideas and expectations about childbirth.

Of course the effects of dominant discourses are not limited to childbirth; they extend to any health or medical issue. In a country that prides itself on being free, Americans as patients are nonetheless often yoked to a single and hierarchically controlled vision of health care. In the United States, health care is equated with biomedicine and with the views that physicians are objective bioscientists and that illnesses and diseases are deviations from a biological norm, have universal features, and have "specific and discoverable causes" (Segal, *Health* 24). Within biomedicine's hierarchy of care, physicians are situated at the top, as heroes of medicine (on "heroic medicine" see Segal, *Health* 24; also see Ehrenreich and English). For example, in the United States, medical procedures and tests are typically *ordered* by physicians. (The verb applies both to the patient and to the health care workers who will perform the procedures or tests.) Contrast this with such procedures and tests being *offered* and discussed both in terms of "professional-expert discourses" and patients' "lay-lifeworld discourses," as Philippa Spoel shows they are, for example, by midwives in Canada ("How Do Midwives Talk with Women?").

In US health care, physicians' authority is typically viewed as the most valid bodily authority, and patients are expected to be compliant to that authority in health care situations. And yet individual women often view and seek childbirth experiences as individual choices, rather than as physician-directed medical events, looking for some degree of separation from the institutional or cultural expectations of modern childbirth. Even women who choose (or "choose") to adhere to the most dominant forms of health discourses make claims. They make arguments. They speak; they write. Melissa Light's creation of a public Facebook page is a recent example of a woman harnessing the space of the Internet to make what I see as a feminist claim—a claim for autonomy from patriarchal medical control of childbirth. Her story provides readers some context for the ways women's birth choices matter, both politically and rhetorically, and for the ways women extend their rhetorical agency by turning to the Internet.

This book honors and explores the rhetorical choices of everyday women—women whose vocations range from stay-at-home mother to lawyer to bus driver[4]—who write birth stories and post them online. These everyday women are using writing and technology to share and understand their experiences, and often as ways to write against/about patriarchal control and institutionalized medicine. This book examines the rhetorical functions of those birth stories and the sites on which they are housed; it examines women's rhetorical choices and influences as birthing women and as writers. It considers the rhetorical choices some of those women made prior to birth in writing birth plans, and it looks at women's agency-making strategies during childbirth, a significant element of many women's reproductive health. This book articulates the rhetorical dimensions of childbirth, showing how terms, definitions, cultural scripts, birth genres (birth plans and birth narratives), online sites, and rhetorical tactics converge.

Birth plans and birth narratives intervene in our society's accepted views of childbirth, sometimes challenging the dominance of medicalized understandings of and beliefs about this event. In *Permanence and Change*, Kenneth Burke lays out the history of belief as a linear progression from magic to religion to science. In the prologue to the 1954 edition, he refines this theory somewhat, suggesting that instead of replacing one another, the three belief systems instead work in tandem (xxv). I see childbirth as a prime example of both Burke's early theory and his revision. To one way of thinking, a quick gloss of childbirth history[5] shows a linear progression that aligns with Burke's early theory. Childbirth in the United States has moved over time, from Europe to the United States, and from magic to religion to science. Early European midwives were associated with "magic," but then "religion" (the Catholic church) sought to control childbirth, prosecuting and persecuting midwives as witches for their use of and association with this "magic." And in time, "science" (which conflates with medicine in this story) replaced "religion" as the primary source of childbirth beliefs; science remains the belief system du jour. Science is credited with developing and supporting childbirth practices in today's hospitals in the United States and much of the West.

Modern Americans' beliefs are overwhelmingly tied to a progress narrative favoring science, but competing belief systems assert themselves both culturally and within individuals. Those competing, simultaneous beliefs reflect Burke's revised theory, which sees these three beliefs—in magic, religion, and science—continuing to play interrelated roles in what could be described as today's childbirth rituals. Women's childbirth choices are also delimited by culture, family, and trust in Western medicine, not to mention by medical insurance.[6]

While Burke's initial explanation of religion replacing magic and science replacing religion suggests a progress narrative, his revised notion provides a more complex acceptance of blended discontinuity, of different beliefs and epistemologies coexisting rather than replacing one another. Women's online birth narratives often show how different, contradictory beliefs coexist, as this excerpt illustrates:

> Around 12 midnight they checked me again. I was at 4 to 5 cm. They said do you want an epidural and I said YES. And see this is the only part I hated about my pregnancy. I was like I'm scared of that epidural and I didn't want it so I was like well I better get it as I can't stand the pain. He stuck me and it didn't hurt at all. I hardly felt it . . . the IV hurt way worse . . . so I definitely recommend an epidural. (Chassie)

Chassie's full caps "YES" in response to the question about an epidural contrasts with her other sentiment: "I'm scared of that epidural and I didn't want it." Her beliefs about the safety or experience of the epidural, or even her need for one, do not emerge as consistent stances; Chassie goes on to say, "I better get it as I can't stand the pain," and she "definitely recommend[s] an epidural." The dominant option of medical assistance with pain prevails, even to the point of advising other women to choose that route, but Chassie's experience of this choice is neither a foregone conclusion nor one she seems to celebrate: "this is the only part I hated about my pregnancy." Conflicting personal beliefs coexist and (re)surface in Chassie's birth narrative.

Online childbirth narratives do more than illustrate the coexistence of conflicting beliefs. They are a material practice that evolves in response to material situations. Birth narratives, birth plans, and online communities and websites devoted to childbirth are all discursive responses, responses we might, following Michel Foucault, call "technologies of the self." For Foucault, technologies of the self "permit individuals to effect by their own means or with the help of others a certain number of operations on their own bodies and souls, thoughts, conduct, and way of being" ("Technologies" 18). Online birth narratives are "technologies of the self," one of the four types of interrelated technologies Foucault delineates: technologies of production, technologies of sign systems, technologies of power, and technologies of the self (18). Childbirth and childbirth writing offer spaces through which we can see these technologies vie for discursive prominence.

To a certain extent, this book is about how women use technologies of the self (for example, birth plans and birth narratives) and of production (such as books and merchandise in a consumer culture) to respond to technologies of sign systems (like pregnancy tests and electronic fetal monitors) and of power (for instance, cultural expectations, hospital hierarchies, and insurance protocols). One issue I explore in this book, then, is how women use technologies of writing to confront, or to claim rhetorical agency over, technologies of birth. Technologies are of course not neutral—they can both solve and create problems, both limit and expand women's voices and choices.

The book focuses on the Internet—a technology that spans each of Foucault's four categories, depending how it is deployed or used—in part because its use is ubiquitous for health information: in 2006, 113 million Americans searched for health information online (Fox). The Internet is a significant source of medical information—both sanctioned and not—and provides a space for women to produce their own everyday rhetorics of health and medicine. This book illuminates the early role of the Internet in shaping both the information women have access to and the everyday rhetorics of health and medicine they produce. I examine how and why modern American women write about childbirth and the work women expect their writing to perform. Rhetorical analysis of birth plans, childbirth and parenting websites, and online birth narratives lays bare the interplay between embodied and educational forms of knowledge, between dominant and niche epistemologies.[7] With an eye on Foucauldian notions of power, I examine the way language, an often unacknowledged player in any childbirth event, affects outcomes, and vice versa, in a self-perpetuating cycle of medical and gender hierarchies.

As with many qualitative research projects, the most important insights emerged in answer to questions I hadn't initially posed. My original aim for this project was to study and understand women's ways of writing childbirth. The consent form for my survey explained this goal in the simplest terms:

> I am researching how and why women write about childbirth. I am looking at birth plans and online birth stories to see what I can learn from them about childbirth practices and how writing may help women understand and deal with childbirth. This survey asks women who have posted online birth stories to answer questions about their childbirth and writing experiences. (appendix A)

I was interested in why and how women wrote online childbirth narratives and birth plans, and I was interested in contributing to understandings of how the Internet—and more specifically, websites devoted to sharing childbirth and parenting information—changed women's expectations, senses of their options, or responses to childbirth. Through reading the completed surveys and working with the data, I discovered answers to those questions, but I also uncovered more questions, questions whose answers speak beyond childbirth.

One question in particular raised through this study was the question of how and to what effect(s) women assert feminist rhetorical agency, or their sense that their words could determine their childbirth experiences. The answer to that question is the book's main argument—that women's individual rhetorical (and material) choices are shaped by Western medicine's dominant discourses, hierarchies, and rhetorical spaces to such an extent that even when women assert rhetorical agency before the fact (via birth plans) or during birth itself, the rhetorical agency they assert is often not equivalent to "success," as is typically understood. While the women in my study didn't necessarily identify as feminists, I claim that women seeking to challenge or express issues with the male-dominated Western medical status quo of modern American hospital births are asserting a rhetorical agency that is undeniably feminist.

The book, then, offers a challenge to the view that individual feminist rhetorical agency necessarily equates with individual control over institutionally situated experiences such as hospital childbirth in the United States. In that sense it suggests a limit to feminist rhetorical agency. Yet I also find that many women seek ways to reclaim rhetorical agency after the fact, via, for example, online childbirth narratives. These assertions illustrate women's abiding urge to establish rhetorical agency and suggest that feminist rhetorical agency cannot be understood solely in terms of success or at a particular moment frozen in time. Feminist rhetorical agency—extended in part by the Internet—can also be understood in terms of women's shaping of events for their own and others' understanding and reassessment across time and space. Close analysis of these women's individual rhetorical acts contributes to theoretical understandings of rhetorical agency, women's writing, and women as patients.

RHETORICAL NEGOTIATIONS, EXPERIENCE, AND STORIES

> After several emotional and upsetting "false alarm" trips to the hospital, I finally went in and whined untill my OB induced me (10 days before my due date. Both of my other children were 2 weeks late and over 8 pounds).
>
> I had left that morning, another false alarm, and teary eyed I cojoled and begged for an induction. I was very surprised. (Rachael)

> The nurse asked me if I wanted an epidural and I said yes. The biggest mistake of my life!! Labor after that became a nightmare. Apparently, they had to drip some fluid into my vein before the anesthesia, which took an eternity—almost an hour of more contractions. At one point I said I had to push and they told me I could not and had to hold on! (Anna)

As a feminist scholar of rhetoric and writing, my interest in childbirth lies not only in women's experiences but also in how women's writings reflect, challenge, or reinscribe various rhetorical and cultural constructions, or cultural scripts, of childbirth. I reveal how women struggle to situate themselves both within and against institutions, medicine, consumer culture, and competing systems of belief, often using language that is itself saturated with those concepts and systems. I argue that these struggles and (shifting) identifications surface as *women's rhetorical negotiations of the complex event of childbirth* through their writing.

Women make these rhetorical negotiations with themselves, with their partners and families, and with their care providers, as the above excerpts from Anna's and Rachael's birth stories show; while women tend to occupy preexisting subject positions to some extent, they also extend beyond those boundaries to create new or seemingly contradictory positions as their knowledge and rhetorical agency shift. Women's personal experience is always at the heart of their rhetorical and material choices—experience is tied up with the birth plans discussed in the first half of this book and the birth narratives that populate the second half. Women's experiences with health and medical information online and offline and with their own bodies, families, and beliefs work together to inform their epistemologies, to frame their birth stories, and to create and recreate their rhetorical negotiations of childbirth.

Women's attempts at fashioning birth experiences and, simultaneously, identities as mothers rely on experience. Experience, though, is at the same time both significant and suspect. As historian Joan W. Scott writes, "Experience is at once always already an interpretation *and* something that needs to be interpreted" (797). And because experience can be shared—translated and interpreted—only through language, experience itself can be understood, broadly speaking, as rhetorical. Further, "what counts as experience is neither self-evident nor straight-forward; it is always contested, and always therefore political" (797). Scott suggests here that experience—because of its very nature—cannot be a foundational source of information. (And indeed, perhaps no foundational source exists, apart from interpretations.) Scott argues that "it is not individuals who have experience, but subjects who are constituted through their experience" (779). It is the inquiry into that subject-constitution that is significant for humanities scholars: the whys and the hows are ultimately more important than the whats.

In the birth plans and stories I examine, I contextualize women's experiences to examine their positioning in relation to institutions and broader cultural structures as part of the analysis. And in my own birth stories, shared in the epilogue, I acknowledge that my position is something of a construct, my choices made as much by "me" as by my positions as a researcher and as a white, overeducated American woman in her early thirties. The ways I exerted (or didn't) rhetorical agency-as-control over my births, and my own rhetorical negotiations of childbirth, are inextricably related to those positions. My choices, like any woman's, are personal; but as Donna Haraway describes with her metaphor of the "bush" of experience, what is personal—an individual woman's choice or experience—also has local and global implications; the local and the global are each also personal and political.

Birth stories, like all stories, organize experience; they make it knowable and memorable. Jerome Bruner suggests that we "cling to narrative models of reality and use them to shape our everyday experiences" (*Making Stories* 7). On these terms, each of the genres treated in the book can also be viewed as a different kind of story, drawing on, sharing, and/or shaping a different kind of experience or knowledge. Birth advice provides a range of stories about what could happen. A birth plan tells the story of what a woman hopes will happen. Hospital protocols and directives from entities like the American Medical Association and the American Congress of Obstetricians and Gynecologists share stories of how and when each character (woman, nurse, doctor, midwife, technology, institution) is expected to act. And, finally, a birth narrative delivers the story of what happened from the author's perspective.

This project relies upon the term *birth stories* as women's stories of their own birth experiences, but it also draws on and resonates with scholarship that defines birth stories differently, such as Mary M. Lay's discussion of midwives' and obstetricians' uses of one another's birth stories to enhance their understandings of their craft, to debate proper procedures and interventions, and, where possible, to find common ground with other practitioners ("Midwives' Birth Stories"; *Rhetoric of Midwifery*). Tess Cosslett, in *Women Writing Childbirth*, analyzes "birth-stories"[8] shared in literature by such authors as

Toni Morrison and Margaret Atwood.[9] She points out that until the twentieth century, childbirth in literature was usually presented from the perspective of attendants or fathers, not from that of the birthing woman (1). Cosslett's analysis begins to recuperate women's missing voices, a recuperation she sets in motion by amplifying the voices of already published authors. I extend this recuperation, applying it to the further submerged voices of everyday women who have not published in the traditional sense but who are everyday writers, women who have written and posted their stories online.[10]

RHETORICS OF BIRTH AS EVERYDAY RHETORICS OF HEALTH AND MEDICINE

> I would only tell them [physicians and nurses] to be a little more concerned about the mother's needs after having major surgery. I think they should have insisted I get some rest that first night. But I guess I could have spoke up as well. My hospital experience was nothing but positive. I've learned that as a patient you need to speak up and take control of your situation. You do have choices. I said no to the many drugs they wanted to give me at various stages. I also avoided strong pain killers and only once requested extra strength Tylenol. (Sandra)

> In response to the recent concerns surrounding VBAC (Vaginal Birth After Cesarean) I wanted to write my birth story and give hope to those wanting to experience a vaginal delivery after a cesarean. My history is long and a little complicated, but it is my own. (Amy)

Online birth stories, along with the birth plans and survey responses examined in this book, are forms of vernacular discourse, to use Gerard Hauser's term. Hauser argues in *Vernacular Voices* that rhetorical scholars must pay attention not only to official discourse but also to discourse produced by everyday citizens, because the interaction between those two discourses reveals how people's opinions are shaped and provides a fuller picture of how people make sense of their shared world, even when they have different understandings and ways of negotiating that world. Online birth stories offer one point of access to everyday women's experiences as women and as patients at one critical stage of their reproductive lives.

Everyday women who write birth stories, like Amy, who teaches sixth grade, make rhetorical choices and seek to have effects on audiences. Inquiry into these women's writing marries two strands of rhetorical knowledge and inquiry: rhetorics of the everyday and rhetorics of health and medicine. Like all forms of rhetoric, the writing is "imbricated with the practical arts of politics and ethics" and "contributes to the perception of material conditions, and indeed at times to their very construction" (Sullivan and Porter 39, 108). Women's everyday childbirth rhetorics not only contribute to the perception of material conditions but are formed by and help form material conditions—and not only of childbirth but more broadly of health and medicine and women's roles in society.

Up to this point, I've alluded to how birth plans and birth narratives can be understood as rhetorical and subject to rhetorical analysis. Let me point now to how I understand rhetoric and its relevance to my inquiry. This project examines *how women use writing to create, manage, and resist various meanings of and experiences with childbirth*, with a triad of verbs borrowed from Martin Nystrand and John Duffy's definition of rhetoric as "the ways that individuals and groups use language to constitute their social realities, and as a medium for creating, managing, or resisting ideological meanings" (ix).

This book explores *how women accept, negotiate, and/or resist various subject positions* in and through their birth writing. In doing so, it follows Karlyn Kohrs Campbell's understanding of rhetorical agency as "the ways in which individuals accept, negotiate, and resist the subject-positions available to them at given moments in a particular culture" (4). Campbell's concepts of negotiation and of qualities of time (*kairos*) resonate readily for this project about childbirth, with its myriad players and unpredictable moments. Further, Michel de Certeau's explanation that "both rhetoric and everyday practices can be defined as internal manipulations of a system—that of language and that of an established order" (24) speaks eloquently to my position that women's childbirth writings should be viewed as everyday rhetorical artifacts.

One reason to illuminate women's birth narratives has to do with their relative absence from dominant conversations in the United States. Rhetorician Krista Ratcliffe has deemed that absence an "exile," exploring the various rhetorical strategies that have conspired to keep women's birth stories silenced ("Bearing Witness" 43). While various birth stories by literary authors have begun to give voice to some birthing women, those voices are few and only relatively recent. Everyday women's stories, while traditionally shared with only a small few, have recently begun to be shared widely with the aid of technology.

Another reason to illuminate and analyze women's birth stories is that these stories are everyday rhetorics of health and medicine: everyday women's writings about their own bodies and experiences within (or outside) the biomedical system. My project connects these women's everyday rhetorics—a concept I extend to include writing that circulates around everyday activities and is available online—with standardized or institutionalized rhetorics of labor. Exploring the rhetorical functions of these stories serves dual feminist and rhetorical aims. This project supports and amplifies the voices of women who have already chosen to speak (write): I surveyed only women who had posted their birth stories, who had taken it upon *themselves* to share their stories, from cesarean section to home birth.

Indispensable to this project is the work of the only other rhetorician who has thus far devoted significant energy to exploring rhetorics of childbirth.[11] In *The Rhetoric of Midwifery*, Mary M. Lay examines the rhetorical power (and lack thereof) of Minnesotan midwives' professional communication. Lay studied both testimony and texts of hearings on the status of lay midwives in that state, who had been serving in an alegal capacity. She writes about the complicated status of traditional, or lay, midwives and certified nurse midwives and explores how the interests of and rhetorical arguments made by these two groups converge and diverge. My project extends Lay's work by bringing a rhetorical lens to everyday women's birthing discourse. While Lay provides insight into the rhetorical context of the work of midwifery and into the rhetorical power and agency of midwives, mine focuses on the rhetorical context of childbirth for birthing women and on the rhetorical power and agency of everyday women in rhetorical spaces online and offline.

METHODS

Because this project connects various fields and types of texts, it draws upon many methods, with rhetorical analysis as the primary methodology. To familiarize myself with women's experiences and discourses, I began by reading hundreds of online birth narratives on five popular childbirth and parenting websites: *Childbirth.org*, *TheLaborofLove.com*, *Plomp.com*, *UnassistedChildbirth.com*, and *BirthStories.com*.[12] I chose 120 narratives in order to have a hearty data set of narratives that spanned the full spectrum of birthing locations, attitudes, and experiences[13] to include in the Institutional Review Board–approved study. I favored stories of first births because first birth stories are based more on educational knowledge than on experiential knowledge; subsequent births are always experienced and usually written about in direct comparison to the embodied experience of the first. The five websites included represent the breadth of those easily accessible online at the time of my study and form the basis for my observations about online birth stories.[14]

After selecting narratives, I emailed a childbirth writing survey (see appendixes A and B) to authors of those stories whose email addresses were provided, with a 25 percent response rate: thirty-four women completed my survey.[15] Of those, seventeen (50 percent of respondents) had written birth plans, and five of those seventeen still had their birth plans and were willing to share them with me.

The survey (see appendix B) offered women open-ended questions and space to describe their experiences, rationales, and expectations for their childbirth writings. I kept most questions open-ended and encouraged responses beyond questions. Gail Hawisher and Patricia Sullivan argue that "a primary goal of feminist research is to empower, to improve the lot of the participants" (180); by providing women a chance to write about their births and birth stories, I hoped to provide that sense of empowerment for participants, and I hope readers will benefit. Respondents took advantage of the space and opportunity to write, sharing ideas and stories now essential to the project. Survey responses are included in my analysis throughout the book, and the birth plans I obtained through the survey provide data for chapters 2 and 3.

Because the survey was online and women had the option to remain anonymous, most women's direct participation in the study was limited to completing the survey. While I initially hoped the survey would be a starting point for further online interaction with respondents, sparking a sort of virtual ethnography, women's responses indicated this was not their priority. A few women requested to read my completed work; I fulfilled those requests by emailing chapters to those women, which marked the end of our communication.

MAPPING CHAPTERS: WHAT LIES AHEAD

The book is organized to mimic a modern American woman's experience of childbirth. Thus it begins with the medical and lay childbirth texts that shape dominant understandings of birth (chapter 1) and then follows an informational/experiential arc of researching birth online and writing a birth plan (chapters 2 and 3) and of giving birth and sharing the story (chapters 4 and 5, as well as the epilogue).

Chapter 1, "Understanding Birth," traces various historical narratives of childbirth in popular and medical texts. It introduces and contrasts the two conflicting grand narratives of childbirth in order to reveal the cultural constraints women and their birth attendants confront as these grand narratives exercise overwhelming force on their epistemologies. The dominant discourses and cultural scripts for birth limit individual women's agency.

Chapters 2 and 3 treat birth plans. "Inventing Birth" connects women's birth plans to the rhetorical canon of invention, exploring how women resist dominant conceptions of childbirth even as they simultaneously reflect other "commonsense" conceptions of the event. The chapter problematizes birth plans' promise of regaining or retaining women's feminist rhetorical agency or control over childbirth. Chapter 3, "Confronting Birth," shows that women giving birth can be positioned as "rhetorically disabled," lacking agency, and that women write birth plans out of an expectation that their spoken voices will not be heard in delivery rooms. While a birth plan's outcome is often influenced more by the rhetorical space of the hospital than by the rhetorical strategies women employ, the birth plan can also empower women.

Chapters 4 and 5 shift the focus to online birth narratives. "Hosting Birth" identifies the key textual, visual, and commercial features of the childbirth and parenting websites included in this study to argue that those websites—and the norms they establish, affirm, or occasionally challenge—affect the extent and distribution of women's rhetorical agency in online birth stories. Chapter 5, "Sharing Birth," reveals that writing and reading online childbirth narratives help women reconcile their childbirth expectations with their experiences and that some women write themselves into positions of rhetorical agency (sometimes retroactively) and/or encourage others to resist the hegemony of Western medicine.

The epilogue examines and challenges assumptions that scholarly work on a topic like childbirth requires or is somehow authorized only by personal experience with the topic, even as it argues that sharing relevant personal experience benefits readers. The epilogue includes autoethnographic accounts of my two home births, accounts that echo features of the birth stories in my study and reveal how this scholarly project influenced those births.

CHAPTER ONE

UNDERSTANDiNG BiRTH

Commonplaces of Modern American Childbirth Advice

> Medicine is not only rhetorical as it is reproduced in published text; it is also rhetorical as a system of norms and values operating discursively in doctor-patient interviews, in hospital corridors, in public debate on health policy, and in the apparatus of disease classifications.
>
> —Judy Segal, *Health and the Rhetoric of Medicine*

Medicine—along with other forms of bodily knowledge—is reproduced through texts and norms, in conversations both private and public. All knowledges are shaped by language, by stories, and by the discursive framing of personal experiences and cultural history. Discursive framing shapes pregnancy and childbirth, too: while there are cultural and individual differences, the majority of birthing women are steeped in and subject to the dominant discourses of their surrounding culture.

This chapter explores the dominant discourses of childbirth in the United States, identifying arguments, tropes, and salient rhetorical features that circulate in a broad range of historical and modern texts. It provides a sketch of American childbirth history that will orient readers for the nuanced investigations into women's childbirth writing and online childbirth information in the chapters that follow. The chapter argues that these dominant discourses create and sustain (sometimes mistaken) beliefs about childbirth and medical progress that dramatically affect US women's roles as agents in childbirth.

To begin to address the dominant discourses surrounding childbirth, let me quickly revisit the story of my being "almost" born in a Volkswagen bus after a camping trip. The story is commonly framed as a tale of danger thwarted by the nick-of-time hospital arrival; this is the story of the medical progress narrative, a grand narrative. While the hospital has only in the last century become the location most commonly associated with childbirth, that institutional site itself is now a trope for childbirth safety. The nick-of-time hospital arrival is a modern story, one that relies on a belief in medical progress over time, a progress narrative that structures history as a story of steady improvements, an epideictic tale of celebration.[1]

The progress narrative is often applied to histories of science and medicine because, as Jeanne Fahnestock shows, when science is "accommodated" for the public, its accommodations are "overwhelmingly epideictic: their main purpose is to celebrate rather than validate" (279). In the context of childbirth, the accommodated epideictic development story goes something like this: ignorance, filth, and death have been replaced—through medical advances—by superior knowledge, sterility, and life. For my mother's story to "work" as a dramatic telling of saved-by-hospital-arrival, both teller and listeners have to accept/expect an overarching medical/scientific progress narrative, in which hospitals (along with physicians and nurses) are cast as saviors whose knowledge and technology provide safe haven. And the story usually works this way, in part because belief in the medical progress narrative is embedded in contemporary American society.

This chapter explains how the medical progress narrative, dominant discourses, and cultural scripts shape contemporary women's choices, including their plans for, experiences of, and writing about childbirth. It also reveals how hospitals, physicians, and nurses came to signify safety for modern American women and demonstrates how medical progress narratives can and have had material effects on birthing women. As an example of a cultural preference for linear progress narratives and of how a dominant belief circulates despite various forms of evidence that refute its veracity, the chapter begins with a brief case study of everyday rhetorics surrounding the history of maternal mortality.

MATERNAL MORTALITY (MIS)INFORMATION

A common theme in both written and oral discussions of childbirth is the perception that historically, childbirth was exceedingly and inherently life-threatening for women and that it is safer now only because of the advent of modern obstetric technologies and methods. In reality childbirth is relatively safe for US mothers now because of improved sanitation, improved access to food, and improved understanding of germs (see Wagner). (The

National Center for Health Statistics reports that the maternal mortality rate for 2003 to be 12.1 per 100,000, or 0.0121 percent.)[2] The idea that, contrasted with today's low rates, dying in childbirth was historically the norm rather than the exception circulates alongside and despite various forms of evidence to the contrary[3] and influences women's understanding of childbirth and the biomedical childbirth system.

Nearly all of the readily available lay childbirth texts offer some statement about how lucky women are to be pregnant in this time period. In *The Girlfriends' Guide to Pregnancy,* author Vicki Iovine asks, "Remember all those episodes on *Bonanza* when the poor women died in childbirth?" (xix), deftly assuming that women's knowledge of the historical dangers of childbirth stem from popular media images.[4] Iovine reassures her audience (filling in reasons based on her beliefs), "You almost never hear about that happening anymore, thanks to God and the American Medical Association" (xix). The Sears' *Birth Book* proclaims, "Gone is the fear of death for baby and mother in childbirth" (15), and the physician's foreword to the unavoidable *What to Expect When You're Expecting* declares, "These are the best years in history to be expecting a baby" (Aubry xx).

Statements like these are part of a culture of enthymematic argument in which claims are based on unstated assumptions or reasons. As Krista Ratcliffe explains, "Unstated *assumptions* not only drive thought, communication, and action, but they also drive the status quo; they hinder change because change is dependent upon changing not just thought and actions but assumptions. Unstated *reasons* drive the status quo because the speaker/writer assumes the reasons to be self-evident" ("In Search" 281). With regard to maternal mortality, the enthymeme can work something like this: A hundred or so years ago, maternal mortality was higher than it is today. A hundred or so years ago, more women gave birth with midwives and at home. Seemingly reasonable conclusion: Maternal mortality rates are lower today because more women give birth in a hospital with physicians than at home with midwives. Or it could go like this: A hundred or so years ago, maternal mortality was higher than it is today. A hundred or so years ago, electronic fetal monitors had not yet been invented. Seemingly reasonable conclusion: Maternal mortality rates are lower today because of electronic fetal monitoring. Or one more: A hundred or so years ago, maternal mortality was higher than it is today. A hundred or so years ago, far fewer women gave birth by cesarean. Seemingly reasonable conclusion: Maternal mortality rates today are lower because of cesarean sections. Missing from each of these is a major premise linking correlation with causation, but the dominance of the medical progress narrative is such that many Americans, even rhetoricians, may uncritically accept these arguments.

Enthymemes in medical progress narratives contribute to a popularly exaggerated sense of historical maternal death rates; maternal mortality stories in popular culture cultivate and perpetuate beliefs about the dangers of childbirth, which exacerbate dominant beliefs about the necessity and function of modern biomedical birth practices. These rhetorics, circulating through different sectors of literate society, help shape our understandings of historical childbirth (in the same way that television and film images shape our perceptions and expectations about current childbirth practices and safety). Several popular books in a variety of genres feature childbed deaths, from Charles Dickens's *Oliver Twist* and Mary Shelley's *Frankenstein* to Chris Bohjalian's *Midwives* (an Oprah's Book Club selection), Gabriel García Márquez's *One Hundred Years of Solitude*, Khaled Hosseini's *The Kite Runner*, George R. R. Martin's *A Game of Thrones*, and J. K. Rowling's Harry Potter series. Movies like the *Star Wars* films and television programs like *Lost* also rely on this trope of mothers who die in childbirth. All of these stories reach disparate but not discrete audiences, and each one (re)invents the idea that death in childbirth itself has been a common, as opposed to a possible but never quite probable, outcome.[5]

In colonial times, the rhetoric surrounding childbirth—from sermons to women's diaries and letters[6]—emphasized fear, danger, and the possibility of death to degrees that far surpassed the risk. These fears may have been "due to cultural and religious factors. Puritan ministers, for example, stressed the likelihood of death in childbirth" (Dye 100). While some scholarly historical accounts (over)emphasize the risk of maternal mortality,[7] historian Nancy Schrom Dye explains that "maternal mortality wasn't very high, at least compared with European rates" (100). The people in North America generally had better health than those in Europe, which contributed doubly to this difference: healthier women had healthier pregnancies and labors, and midwives had less need to interfere with their labors, thus lessening the chances of iatrogenic (treatment-caused) problems.[8]

Beyond popular texts and histories, even conventional, officially sanctioned sources of information available online can contribute to present-day misperceptions about historical maternal mortality. One such powerful and respected source in our society is the Centers for Disease Control (CDC) website, which offers a confusing picture of the available historical evidence:

> Maternal mortality rates were highest in this [the twentieth] century during 1900–1930. Poor obstetric education and delivery practices were mainly responsible for the high numbers of maternal deaths, most of which were preventable. Obstetrics as a specialty was shunned by many physicians, and obstetric care was provided by poorly trained or untrained medical practitioners. Most births occurred at home with the assistance of midwives or general practitioners. Inappropriate and excessive surgical and obstetric interventions (e.g., induction of labor, use of forceps, episiotomy, and cesarean deliveries) were common and increased during the 1920s. ("Achievements")

The CDC passage's conflation of "poor obstetric education" with "delivery practices," followed by the (also true) statement that most births were home births attended by midwives or general practitioners, could readily be interpreted as suggesting that the midwives who attended home births were those with the poor education whose delivery practices caused deaths. The available data, though, provide a somewhat different picture. Namely, the "inappropriate and excessive surgical and obstetric interventions" that were largely responsible for the preventable deaths were most often made by physicians—particularly by physicians working in hospitals—not by midwives catching babies at home ("Achievements").

The CDC's presentation of information makes misinterpretations of the data nearly inevitable, and these misinterpretations fit with present-day biases and expectations mired in progress-narrative belief patterns. My analysis of this passage provides one small example of how even agreed-upon information, depending on how it is written and circulated, can contribute to a heightened sense of the dangers of childbirth in history—beliefs that have material and economic consequences for childbirth perceptions and practices today. To consumers of such information, hospitals and physicians can come to automatically and uncritically signify safety, affecting women's childbirth choices, experiences, and childbirth writing.

PROGRESS NARRATIVES: PROBLEMS WITH THEIR DOMINANCE

The dominance of the progress narrative can have real and dangerous effects for women, as one tale from early American history illustrates well. In the eighteenth and nineteenth centuries, both American and European maternal mortality rates increased dramatically. This increase happened just as physicians were beginning to attend to births alongside or instead of midwives. We now know that many of these deaths were caused by "puerperal fever." (Readers may notice that my phrasing there, "we now know," fits with and contributes to a medical progress narrative arc.) As Judith Rooks explains in *Midwifery and Childbirth in America*, puerperal fever was often spread by "infectious agents transmitted to the mother on the hands of the person who assisted the delivery" (25). Rooks goes on to explain that "it was easy to blame [the deaths on] the midwives, who had no formal training. In fact, doctors, who conducted autopsies and took care of patients with communicable diseases, were much more likely to be at fault" (25). A few midwives, and doctors such as Oliver Wendell Holmes in the United States and Ignaz Philipp Semmelweis in Vienna, suggested at the time that birth attendants were somehow contributing to the deaths (see Rich 153–55), but for decades physicians were resistant to this explanation of the cause of puerperal fever.

Because of their enculturation to the medical progress narrative, most physicians could not see evidence that belied their image of themselves as superior caregivers, and so they unwittingly *caused* death after death. Meanwhile, as Adrienne Rich explains in *Of Woman Born*,

> the potential sources of the disease went unexplored, and women continued to die—not from giving birth, but from acute streptococcal infection of the uterus, *in no way inevitably linked with the birth process.* It killed one Mary Wollstonecraft, of whom we know, and thousands of women of whom we know nothing. . . . And the specter of death, larger than ever before in the history of maternity, darkened the spirit in which any woman came to term. (153; my emphasis)

As doctors, and as gentlemen, male physicians of the era thought their hands were clean, literally and metaphorically (Cutter and Viets; Rich). Physicians were blind to and dismissive of even the possibility that they could be contributing to maternal deaths.

The story of puerperal fever, with physicians as unwitting "bad guys" who ignored evidence of negative effects of their practices, may appear to contradict the powerful medical progress narrative, and yet it can easily be framed to support it: doctors eventually discovered the error of their ways, began washing their hands between their varied duties (such as attending a birth after conducting an autopsy), and—presto!—maternal mortality decreased. Told this way, it becomes a story of male physicians gaining knowledge through the accepted practice of trial and error. Framed this way, the story of puerperal fever appears as a strange anomaly in the larger tale of medical progress. The implication is that as time passes, new and better knowledge, practices, and practitioners simply and irrevocably replace or improve upon older (and in this model inferior) knowledges, practices, and practitioners.

That notion of medical progress carries continuing challenges and dangers, as rhetorician Joseph Dumit illustrates. Dumit relays the story of his wife's ectopic pregnancy, a dangerously misimplanted embryo that went undiagnosed for weeks despite numerous doctor visits and ultrasounds interpreted by multiple physicians. Sylvia Sensiper was a "DES daughter." (DES, or diethylstilbestrol, was commonly prescribed to women as a miscarriage preventative from 1938 through 1975 [Dumit and Sensiper 219]. The drug did prevent miscarriage but had unanticipated effects on the reproductive functions of the *children* of the women who took it. These children grow up suffering from reproductive abnormalities ranging from increased risk of cancer to misshapen reproductive organs to infertility.) Because of Sensiper's in-utero exposure to this drug and her resultant uterine abnormalities, her chances of ectopic pregnancy were 13.5 times higher than for the general population (214). Yet her physicians, though made aware of her status, seemed to ignore it. In an effort to understand why his wife's physicians failed to notice important evidence, leading to a life-threatening misdiagnosis, Dumit traced DES information in physicians' textbooks and handbooks.

Dumit found that medical textbooks offer consistent, accurate, and fairly complete information about DES but that medical *handbooks* (which are smaller, more concise, and more easily and regularly referenced by busy practicing physicians) often fail to include in-utero exposure to DES as a risk factor for ectopic pregnancy. The handbooks include no indications of any required special care and sometimes even omit DES altogether. This omission, Dumit asserts, leads physicians to believe DES to be a problem of the past, a belief instilled or upheld by the ways information about DES and its multigenerational effects (or any medical or health facts) circulate or, more pointedly in this case, cease to circulate.

Dumit's study demonstrates that medicine does not always use its own best knowledge and evidence in practice, for a variety of reasons, one of which is a prevailing, if often invisible, expectation that medicine's progress is consistent and uncomplicatedly good. Believing that knowledge simply builds upon itself over time produces uncritical acceptance of new procedures and technologies along with uncritical dismissal of older procedures and technologies, and it impedes both lay and medical people in their understandings of childbirth (or of any medical or health event).

The progress narrative is the most common grand narrative, but its counterpoint, the decline narrative, suggests that instead of improving over time, childbirth instead devolved over time. The decline narrative tells the story of childbirth shifting from what once was a woman-centered, easy and/or empowering, largely safe endeavor to one that is machine-centered, demeaning, and both physically and emotionally unsafe. In this view, birth has moved from idyllic to traumatic. A quick visual reference to each narrative can be found in Monty Python's *The Meaning of Life*, where viewers see the contrast between a woman standing, singing, and pinning up laundry while giving birth to her umpteenth child, and another woman giving birth in hospital. The hospitalized woman, surrounded by multiple masked physicians and the "machine that goes 'Ping!,'" asks what she can do and is told she is "not qualified" to do anything.

In the Monty Python sketch, one finds ready access to three critical elements of childbirth, the choice, availability, or assumptions of which dramatically affect women's childbirth experiences. These three are location, attendants, and support, and each shows up prominently in all historical, medical, and lay literatures. In the next two sections I explore these three always-important aspects of childbirth to examine how the dominant discourses of childbirth function in and through them; location and attendant are so interrelated for American childbirth that I treat them together.

LOCATION AND ATTENDANTS: SHIFTING CONTROL

> "Medicalized" childbirth is relatively new, a product of the twentieth century. Even though we have come to accept it as typical, the historical record is very clear on how recently a phenomenon it is for physicians to be in control of labor and delivery and for women to bow to their expertise. (Judith Leavitt, *Make Room for Daddy*, 21–22)

> My first "birth" experience . . . turned into a cataclysmic disaster at the hospital, where my baby son, Hans, was cut out of and taken from me via Caesarean section. The general anesthesia had not yet taken

> effect when the surgeon began slicing into my belly. It took me years to sort through it all and figure out and learn what really happened and why. . . . I totally misunderstood the concepts of "taking responsibility for" and "owning" one's own pregnancy and birth experience. I had no idea what birth was. Granted, it was a far cry from going to an OB and mindlessly assuming a hospital "delivery," but you see, it ended up the same way. (Corey)

> I dreamed of delivering my own baby, unassisted since I first became aware of where babies come from. I really could not fathom the idea of being watched by strangers for such an intimate act. (Stacy)

In terms of location and birth attendants, the progress narrative in the United States causes physicians and hospitals to be perceived as the safest options. These options are also the default for most American women, having almost entirely replaced the previous default of midwives and home birth. It wasn't always thus, of course.

Childbirth was an all-woman event for most of human history in most cultures. Women exclusively attended and controlled birth in Europe until the sixteenth century and the majority of births through the nineteenth century (Arney; Brodsky; Edwards and Waldorf; Leavitt, *Brought to Bed* and *Make Room*; Wertz and Wertz). Power, as Judith Leavitt has shown in *Brought to Bed*, her definitive history of American women's roles in childbirth from 1750 to 1950, historically rested with women—and not with a single woman but with a group of women. The woman giving birth, the women friends and family invited to attend the birth, and the woman serving as a midwife determined together how each woman's labor would be handled.

When male physicians began to be invited into women's homes for their labors in the 1760s (Leavitt, *Brought to Bed*), their voices did not, as modern Americans might assume, supersede the women's voices. In the home, even with a male physician present, agency over the birth continued to be distributed among the birthing woman, her social coterie, and midwife. Women "had no intention at that time to give over decision-making authority to doctors" (Leavitt, *Make Room* 24). Doctors attending home births learned to work within the home domain, which was not theirs: "Doctors could offer advice, but they did not have the freedom of action in women's homes that they later achieved in hospitals" (26). Richard W. Wertz and Dorothy C. Wertz suggest that physicians attending home births in the nineteenth century chafed under the watch of many women and "were inclined to urge the removal" of all but a "nurse or friend who would obey the doctor's orders" (5). Until birth moved to the hospital, though, physicians could not dictate the number or type of people present for a birth or any of the circumstances of birth.

In 1910 physicians and midwives attended equal numbers of births in the United States, but by 1930 midwives attended only 15 percent (Leavitt, *Brought to Bed*). Hospital births (which meant physician-attended births) accounted for 37 percent of births in 1936; 55 percent of births by 1940; and 90 percent of births by 1951 (Brodsky 132). Today approximately 99 percent of US births take place in hospitals, the vast majority with physicians attending. Nurse-midwives attend only 7 percent of hospital births. Only 0.5 percent—half of one percent—of all births are midwife-attended home births (Martin et al., "Births: Final Data for 2006" 67).[9] This shift in attendants and location was swift, but not smooth.

Based on the progress narrative, one would expect that in the early 1900s, once the causes of puerperal fever were known and antiseptic standards modern readers would recognize were in place, hospital birth would have become significantly safer for women. And yet a 2006 *New Yorker* story reveals that

> in 1933 the New York Academy of Medicine published a shocking study of 2,041 maternal deaths in childbirth. At least two-thirds, the investigators found, were preventable. There had been no improvement in death rates for mothers in the preceding two decades; newborn deaths from birth injuries had actually increased. Hospital care brought no advantages; mothers were better off delivering at home. The investigators were appalled to find that many physicians simply didn't know what they were doing: they missed clear signs of hemorrhagic shock and other treatable conditions, violated basic antiseptic standards, tore and infected women with misapplied forceps. The White House followed with a similar national report. Doctors may have had the right tools, but midwives without them did better. (Gawande)

The study was shocking, of course, because it belied expectations of progress in health and safety. And even though birth's shift to hospitals and physicians actually *increased* maternal mortality for decades, long after the discovery of the causes of puerperal fever, that shift, from home to hospital and midwife to physician, nonetheless continued.

Reasons for this shift include the rise of the automobile and increased number of hospitals, along with lower birth rates, which combined to make hospital deliveries by physicians more feasible than in earlier times. Further, the move to hospital birth reflected women's choice. As Phyllis Brodsky, an obstetric nurse turned childbirth educator and author, explains, "Women sought the sanctuary of hospitals because they believed that they would be safer there than in their own homes" (132). In addition, women believed hospital birth could provide respite from pain that home birth couldn't. For example, women lobbied for access to "twilight sleep," which required hospitalization (Litoff; Leavitt, *Brought to Bed*). Judith Leavitt casts this shift as a "feminist vein"—women working on their own and together, hoping to improve their childbirth experiences—with unintended consequences. Twilight sleep, induced by the drug scopolamine, was advertised as providing pain-free childbirth; instead, Leavitt explains, it caused women to *forget* the pain of labor but also resulted in a lack of emotional and physical control during labor, which led to questionable hospital responses, such as tying laboring women to their beds with lambskins (which left no marks).

Leavitt notes that by 1950, women's own choices had resulted in near-complete medical dominance over childbirth. Brodsky reveals that "in the early and middle years of the twentieth century, women . . . were afraid to deal with any pain, willingly submitting their bodies to their physicians without questioning" (8). Already the progress narrative and the newly dominant cultural script of medicalized hospital birth had replaced the previous cultural script for social childbirth in the home: women "had no idea that childbirth could be conducted differently than it was at the time" (8).

In the space of a century, women's labors shifted from being entirely in multiple women's control in the home to being nearly entirely controlled by physicians (and the nurses whom physicians controlled). In *Reclaiming Birth*, Margot Edwards and Mary Waldorf offer unsettling data about the control that physicians and nurses exerted over women's births in the early to mid-twentieth century, relating the story of the *Ladies' Home Journal* receiving a "flood of letters" in response to an unsigned letter sent by a registered nurse in 1958 detailing "cruelty she had witnessed on maternity wards" (55). Women wrote of feeling hostility rather than the expected kindness from nurses. Women wrote of being left to labor alone for hours, or overnight, while tied up with leather straps. Women wrote of nurses holding or strapping their legs together when it was time to push because physicians had not arrived. (The latter stories appear in contemporary online birth stories as well.) Physicians consulted at the time suggested there was no medical reason to delay imminent births in this manner but explained that nurses "could not be blamed because they had to carry out orders or lose their positions, no matter what their own judgment of the situation might be" (56). The control of physicians in hospital births far exceeded any individual's control in home birth.

In this shift of births to hospitals and physicians' care, midwives were left behind, despite the fact that midwives' care was generally more comprehensive, less expensive, and at least as safe as physicians' care. Perceptions of midwives' care changed as women increasingly believed in the benefits of medical technologies, such as twilight sleep, available only in hospitals and with physicians. Various societal changes put pressure on childbirth choices, contributing to changes in dominant American childbirth culture that persist today.[10]

Between the eighteenth and twentieth centuries, increased beliefs in "science," shifting gender roles, changing attitudes toward and methods of providing pain relief, and changes in women's decision-making power all contributed to changes in childbirth location and attendants (Leavitt, *Brought to Bed*). As Americans increasingly believed in sciences and specialized knowledge, issues of race, class, culture, gender, and literacy became relevant to childbirth choices as well. Midwives were stereotyped as uneducated, dirty, and limited in part because they were usually of lower classes and often were immigrants.

The medical progress narrative, which relies in part on stereotyping and scapegoating midwives, supersedes and excludes other historical frames in part because histories tend to rely on published accounts, which privilege those of higher social class. To write and publish, of course, requires literacy, means, and time, requirements generally more available to men than to women and certainly more available to literate, native-born men. Although female midwives did publish (see Lay; Litoff), they were much less likely than male physicians or "male midwives" (Cutter and Viets) to do so, with the result that much of the history of childbirth relies on accounts by men. Decline narratives of childbirth history, such as those offered by second-wave feminists, explicitly work against tales that overrely on men's published work.

Barbara Ehrenreich and Dierdre English, for example, rely on texts by women in their efforts to avoid what they see as biased information from "the educated elite" (260). Ehrenreich and English explain the shift from midwife to physician and home to hospital in terms of a broader shift from home health care generally provided by women to professionalized health care offered by men (at significant cost), revealing reasons such as a historical conflation between witches and midwives and women healers and such women being stereotyped negatively by men in order to lessen their significance. Ehrenreich and English frame the history of healing, broadly, as a systematic, deliberate replacement of women healers by men, "an active *takeover* by male professionals" (4). The term "professionals" is significant.

Professionalization requires that members of a group take responsibility for their own training (Borst). Unlike physicians, midwives neither sought nor gained control of their own training programs. Midwifery also had different prerequisites than medicine's: midwives were expected to have bodily experience—to be married and to have had children themselves. Many practicing midwives had children at home. Because their work supplemented, rather than supplied, their livelihood, unlike the work of physicians, midwives saw little reason to actively professionalize. As a result, physicians professionalized and gained patients and trust, while midwives didn't, losing both.

A decline narrative suggests that men (church leaders, male midwives, or physicians) deliberately wrested control of childbirth from female attendants, to the detriment of birthing women. As Suzanne Arms tells it in *Immaculate Deception*:

> There is no doubt that the history of childbirth can be viewed as a gradual attempt by man to extricate the process of birth from woman and call it his own. Indeed, some anthropologists and radical feminists believe that man has always been threatened by woman's exclusive power in childbirth, and that by placing his strength and intelligence against her docility and instinct he "won" an authoritarian role in society. (21)

Ironically, though, women's own early feminist efforts to control childbirth, which ranged over time from keeping labor in the home controlled by women to seeking out physicians to advocating for hospital births and anesthesia, do not fit into this decline narrative.

Women successfully asserted feminist rhetorical agency; they obtained their desired access to physicians and hospitals. As Judith Leavitt reveals, "Men did not make significant changes in women's birth experiences *unless and until women invited them to*" (*Brought to Bed* 15; emphasis in original). Leavitt's work recuperates women as powerful contributors to, rather than passive victims of, change, complicating the decline narrative perspective. Further, while physicians' concerns about their livelihoods did lead to their denouncing midwives, that wasn't the only reason midwives fell out of favor. Criticism of midwives reflecting the "anti-immigrant and anti-Negro prejudices of the period" also came from the public (Litoff 77). Thus, prejudice, along with gendered and classed access to literacy and professionalization, contributed to midwives' diminished roles in childbirth.

As physicians professionalized, training themselves and writing textbooks, the medical progress narrative became further sedimented in medical textbooks, which emphasize progress and can deride past knowledge. *Williams Obstetrics*, the gold standard for obstetrical training, serves as a primary example. As with all textbooks, new editions posit their superiority over the last. Authors of the 1966 version of *Williams Obstetrics* explain: "From the viewpoint of safer care during labor, the outstanding advance of the past 25 years has been the great increase in the proportion of hospital deliveries" (Eastman and Hellman 9). The language suggests an economic, industrial agenda. The authors state matter-of-factly that "hospital births not only mean better facilities, but imply care by physicians" (9).[11] Implicit here are two beliefs: that care by physicians is superior, and that birth in a hospital is inherently better than in other locations. These implicit beliefs are also, of course, at play in the "nick-of-time" version of my mother's birth story and continue to inform Americans' childbirth beliefs. These dominant narratives train us as readers and information consumers, inculcating particular beliefs that diminish our abilities to critically examine not only our histories but also our present situations.

CHILDBIRTH SUPPORT: TECHNOLOGICAL AND/OR SOCIAL

> [T]he OB got called in and checked the heartbeat, then said the baby had to be out now! He decided to use forceps, there wasnt any time! The foot-stirrups were put in place, I got a catheter (didnt hurt), a 4th-degree episiotomy (no anestetics, it hurt for a moment), he put in the forceps (no anestetics either, so yes, that hurt a lot!) and pulled our daughter into this world! (Susan)

> I just "let it happen." My girl friend asked what I wanted her to do, I requested that she just pray, aloud! She did, it was very nice! My husband wiped my brow and offered great words of love. I remember telling my

> midwife to "get her elbows out of me." "I'm sitting on the couch behind you watching, but not touching you" she replied. I often yelled her name for reassurance, she'd say "you're doing great, you're so strong"! (Sydney's mother)

Perhaps the best-known form of childbirth support is the forceps, a form of technological support that also happens to have a rather interesting/infamous history. Adrienne Rich explains: "The history of the forceps is a peculiar one, involving three male generations of a family, the commercial exploitation of a scientific invention, and the effective displacement of the midwife through a male monopoly of that invention" (142). Designed in the late 1500s by the Chamberlen brothers, the tool, referred to as "their Secret" (143), was used in difficult births. The Chamberlens, though, kept "their Secret" just that.

The Chamberlens asserted rights to the tool as what we might today call intellectual property, keeping it an industry secret in part by hiding it and chiming bells while it was used, a choice Rich excoriates: "The men who developed the forceps, symbol of the art of the obstetrician, were profiteers" (144). The forceps remained a family secret for three generations, a choice midwives of the era could not understand. Midwives were inclined to share knowledges and tools that would help women; believing the forceps were beneficial, they wanted access but were denied it. (Midwives' lack of access to forceps, even after the Chamberlen monopoly ended, contributed to their lack of professionalization, as examined above.)

As a story of a technology believed to provide only benefits to women and babies, the forceps history fits into a progress narrative. As a story of a technology and its benefits being denied to midwives, forceps history becomes more complicated. And when the dangers associated with forceps deliveries are taken into consideration, the picture becomes muddier still. And yet the prominence of and belief in the tool has been pervasive over time. What is significant for this chapter is the widespread belief that new technologies (of which forceps is one example) always, or even typically, improve birth experiences and outcomes. It is worth noting that while forceps did allow for safe deliveries of some babies who might otherwise not have survived, they also often caused—and can still cause—life-threatening or life-ending injuries to both mothers and babies. The tool came with benefits but also risks.[12]

As with other aspects of modern life, the application of a wide range of technologies to childbirth has increased and normalized over time. These technologies provide (or are meant to provide) support of one kind or another to pregnant and birthing women—for pain relief, pharmaceuticals and spinal blocks; for various diagnoses and determining gestational dates, ultrasounds; for checking the baby's heartbeat, electronic fetal monitors; for delivery problems, forceps or vacuum extractors or now, most commonly, C-sections. Non-technological support exists, too, in the form of social, physical, and emotional assistance with childbirth. These forms have come in and out of favor over time and with different populations (see Arms; Cassidy; Gaskin, *Ina May's Guide*; Mitford; Taylor) but broadly speaking have remained the primary forms of support in home-birth situations and are more common in midwife-attended hospital births, while technological forms tend to dominate in physician-attended hospital births.[13]

Support is one way to examine and explain how physicians' care came to differ from that of midwives. Midwives might simply be "with women," which is what "midwife" means; midwives would participate in "social childbirth" alongside a woman's neighbors and friends (Wertz and Wertz). Once birth shifted to hospitals, women "lost their social, supportive network" of midwife and female friends (Brodsky 132). Physicians were not expected to wait around for hours-long or days-long labors. Women thought nurses would stay with them and fill the supportive role, "but it didn't happen. The nurses were too busy following doctors' orders [and] monitoring their patients. . . . [They] didn't have time to provide comfort of tender loving care to their patients. Medication was the answer to these needs" (132). That support was critical. Modern studies show a marked benefit in having nonmedical women attend births, whether as female friends offering support or in the form of doulas: doulas are paid to provide social, physical, and emotional support to birthing and postpartum women (see England and Horowitz). Doulas provide the constant "being with" support that neither nursing staff nor hospital-based midwives can typically provide. According to Pam England and Rob Horowitz, the presence of doulas leads to shorter labors and significantly reduces epidurals, augmentation with Pitocin, Cesarean births, and forceps births. These benefits seem to result from a combination of continuity of care, one-on-one support throughout labor, a partner freed up to advocate for the birthing woman, and the doula herself acting as an advocate for the birthing woman.

Physicians have never been expected to simply "be with" patients. Historically, physicians, because they dealt with conditions besides childbirth and did so using medicines and particular actions—like bloodletting—were expected to "do something" when attending women's labors, not to wait or emotionally support women. The expectation that physicians act has continued as physicians have become more specialized and more learned in and focused on deviations from what is perceived as normal—a biomedical view and a tradition that echoes the Chamberlens being called for "difficult births." With these changes, women became sites, or objects, of childbirth, while physicians and technologies became childbirth's agents.

Expectations that physicians *perform* led to practices that sometimes hampered rather than helped birth, and yet every successful physician-attended birth, whether because of or in spite of interventions, began to be credited to the doctor's skill. Various economic and social factors led to the increased acceptance of and demand for scientific and technological solutions to health care problems over traditional, "natural," often home-controlled remedies (Wertz and Wertz).

THE ELECTRONIC FETAL MONITOR: OBSTETRIC "SUPPORT" GONE WRONG

Recall Atul Gawande's *New Yorker* story above about problems with childbirth and maternal mortality in the 1930s. The last line of that excerpt, "Doctors may have had the right tools, but midwives without them did better," even while castigating the mistakes of the physicians, suggests that obstetric tools themselves are "right." And yet even Gawande, a physician—a surgeon, in fact—finds certain obstetric tools problematic at best. Gawande also points out that obstetricians are notorious for ignoring research findings and for applying tools that have been proven to be more damaging than useful. He writes:

> Obstetricians did few randomized trials, and when they did they ignored the results. Careful studies have found that *fetal heart monitors provide no added benefit over having nurses simply listen to the baby's heart rate hourly.* In fact, their use seems to increase unnecessary Cesarean sections, because slight abnormalities in the tracings make everyone nervous about waiting for vaginal delivery. Nonetheless, they are used in nearly all hospital deliveries.[14]

Gawande is not alone in pointing to the electronic fetal monitor as a specific example of a gap between obstetricians' uses of technologies and the data about those technologies. Several sources decry a mismatch between obstetric knowledge and practice and an overreliance on ineffective technologies (Goer; Wagner). Sociologist William Ray Arney, in *Power and the Profession of Obstetrics*, partly attributes that problem to obstetrics' interest in "monitoring" pregnancy and birth. Surveillance also, of course, has dramatic effects on pregnant women's actions and interactions with physicians (Foucault, *Discipline*). Of the modern monitoring technologies, the electronic fetal monitor is a primary example.

While the monitor seems to solve a practical problem of how to listen to the fetal heartbeat, a seeming technological advance, it fails to solve what Arney calls "the theoretical problem—what to listen for," and how to interpret and act on those results (102). Arney explains that "using the same body of evidence but speaking from different perspectives and representing different interests, women, the government, and certain obstetricians have questioned the efficacy and safety of monitoring" (106). He goes on to describe how the meaning of terms like "fetal distress" has become more complicated and contested since the advent of technologies like the electronic fetal monitor—far more fetuses are perceived to be in distress than prior to the use of the monitor, but outcomes have not improved since its introduction, perhaps in part because monitors impede physicians' and nurses' abilities to notice and support their patients over the monitor's data about their patient. Brodsky describes witnessing

> busy nurses entering their patients' rooms briefly to study the monitor strip and make notes, but spend[ing] only a few minutes conversing with and comforting their patients. Nurses and doctors tend to get caught up in evaluating the enormous amount of data, trouble-shooting malfunctioning equipment, sacrificing precious time spent with their patients, and "may overlook the subtle, human cues that something is amiss." (165)

While obstetrics has taken "monitoring" as one of its primary tasks, some of the practices associated with monitoring turn out to have no benefit and to sometimes instead do harm. Electronic fetal monitoring increases the number of C-sections without resulting in better outcomes for mother or baby; the only demonstrated outcome of that type of monitoring is more surgeries. Modern Americans tend to believe that more data—a quantitative approach—is better, so if a technology can provide more data, the data should be collected and used. What we see with this case, however, is that a noncontinuous qualitative-quantitative approach—nurses listening manually each hour, for example—has better outcomes. And despite this knowledge, in practice (as measured in 2002) electronic fetal monitors are used in 93 percent of births, while the evidence-based recommendation is 0 percent (Wagner 51). The difference between 93 percent and 0 percent is quite stark and hints at how certain practices and beliefs in medicine persist, to women's detriment, in part because of a medical progress narrative. It also illustrates the abiding control physicians exert over childbirth.

Persistent belief in a technology like electronic fetal monitoring—despite significant evidence against its usefulness—is mired in an assumption of technological progress over time. This assumption carries with it a presumption of approaching perfection: it helps to fuel expectations not only for a reduction of "natural" risks but for an absence of them; it helps to fuel expectations that medicine or a physician is, can, or should be perfect. It also helps to fuel a culture of litigation surrounding even the perception of medical error. And expectations of perfection by medical management of childbirth lead to certain measures of success being accepted while others measures of success are disregarded. For example, Gawande explains that obstetricians are trained to perform C-sections, a surgery they can "perfect"; they are no longer trained to employ more nuanced, nonsurgical solutions, in part because belief in surgery's perfection limits litigation potential, and surgery is seen as the final and best action a physician can take. And yet as Gawande and a chorus of others have noted, C-sections are often not medically warranted and have a host of negative side effects, such as higher childbirth costs, reductions in successful breast-feeding rates, increased risk of postpartum depression, increased risks for future C-sections, and increased maternal mortality rates (see, for example, Cassidy; Goer; Kitzinger; Wagner). (For more on the rhetorical force of C-sections, see Hensley Owens, "Reviews and Reactions").

SHIFTING PARADIGMS, DISCARDED KNOWLEDGE

Certainly in the United States a change not unlike a paradigm shift has occurred, one that began 150 years ago and is now all but complete: for the vast majority of American women, childbirth has shifted from an event of the home, attended by women trained and untrained, to an event of the hospital, attended by physicians. The change is both practical and theoretical, and exceptions to it are incredibly small. This paradigm shift brings with it attendant expectations of progress, even though, as David J. Hess explains, "a paradigm shift or large theoretical change is not necessarily unequivocally progressive" (25). Thomas Kuhn points out that replacing one theory with another means that elements of the previous are discarded, but he also notes that "out-of-date theories are not in principle unscientific because they have been discarded. That choice, however, makes it difficult to see scientific development as a process of accretion" (2–3).

With any paradigm shift, new knowledge comes to *replace*—not just add to—old. As this replacement occurs, some knowledge, however useful or accurate, is inevitably lost; this loss has been called "Kuhn loss" (Hess 25). The concept of the "Kuhn loss" is significant in understanding childbirth histories, particularly in reconciling the progress with the decline narratives. Those who accept a progress narrative—which would include most contemporary Americans, given our nearly universal childbirth choices with anesthesia and the latest technology readily available "just in case"—necessarily deduce that old knowledge is inferior. To most Americans, a loss of "old" knowledge seems, then, not only unproblematic but beneficial. These beliefs circumscribe women's childbirth choices.

On the opposite end of the spectrum, those who accept a decline narrative, rejecting the dominant progress narrative, are likely to romanticize older knowledge, dismissing actual technological, pharmaceutical, or procedural progress. While the simpler historical narratives tend to be favored, we stand to benefit from more complex understandings. We might seek to avoid the Kuhn loss: for example, we know we are losing knowledge and techniques that midwives have employed for centuries to alleviate problems that today's physicians, as Gawande notes, are trained to solve only by performing C-sections, a major surgery. We might seek to avoid losing midwifery's *phronesis*, or "practical wisdom," blending care and theory, to obstetrics' perfection-focused *techne*, instead looking for ways to better blend the two. The idea of perfection, as applied in childbirth, converts the practice of obstetrics from craft to industry and, in doing so, affects women's experiences as they are positioned within the realm of obstetrics and the medical progress narrative that guides their choices. And yet adhering to any set of dominant beliefs can hinder scholars, physicians, and birthing women.

The CDC reports that in 2006, 99.09 percent of US births took place in hospitals, and 91.4 percent of all births were attended by physicians (Martin et al., "Births: Final Data for 2006" 67). Physician-attended hospital births are the obvious norm. Yet despite Americans' overwhelming adherence to the medical progress narrative, illustrated in part by such statistics, some women do make nondominant choices. Some women (7.1 percent in 2006) choose certified nurse midwives as attendants for their hospital births, an option covered by many insurance plans (Martin et al., "Births: Final Data for 2006"). And a small percentage of women give birth beyond hospital walls in birthing centers (0.2 percent) or at home with alternative care providers, such as certified professional midwives or other lay midwives (0.5 percent), often doing so alegally or illegally and paying out-of-pocket because childbirth laws and insurance approvals are themselves yoked to medical discourse.

Women who make nondominant location choices pose both rhetorical and material challenges to childbirth's medical progress narrative.[15] Others present such challenges within the hospital. As consumers of childbirth services, some women discover that the care offered in hospitals does not match their expectations or ideals. Some accept the dominant location and/or dominant care provider but write birth plans in an effort to assert rhetorical agency and to intervene in industrial and legally and technologically bound hospital practices.

The next chapter, "Inventing Birth," examines birth plans and online birth plan advice. Birth plans attempt to guide attendants of hospital labors; the genre, then, embraces or accepts such dominant aspects of childbirth as the location of the hospital but simultaneously resists such dominant aspects as the role of attendants and technological interventions within that space. I show that modern American women writing birth plans attempt to fashion birth experiences for themselves that at once rely upon and challenge childbirth's dominant discourses, commonplace beliefs, and cultural scripts.

CHAPTER TWO

INVENTiNG BiRTH

Rhetorics of Control and Resistance

Bodily control and discipline are valued in modern Western culture.
—Lynda Birke, *Feminism and the Biological Body*

The genre of the birth plan is relatively new and has fairly explicit rhetorical intentions: women write birth plans to claim agency, to some extent, over the circumstances of labor and delivery. As a document written by laypeople and addressed to medical staff,[1] a birth plan is an example of what I am describing as everyday rhetorics of health and medicine. Its language, crafted by ordinary, everyday people, is infused with and responds to dominant health and medical discourses and practices while it simultaneously asserts rhetorical agency over those discourse and practices. Birth plans typically express hopes for a birth with limited medical influence; their very existence relies upon and reflects a woman's knowledge of and desire to avoid or minimize the effects of hospital protocols, technologies, or interventions. The birth plan anticipates a certain level of control over what many see as a largely uncontrollable event.

Birth plans and birth plan advice are forms of rhetoric in the sense that they create, manage, and resist ideological meanings of childbirth in our society.[2] This chapter demonstrates how websites offering birth plan advice reflect and shape collective and individual concerns about modern American childbirth. Further, the chapter argues that the authors of online birth plan advice exhort women to assert feminist rhetorical agency over their births without recognizing that their advice can also inadvertently thwart opportunities for the success of those assertions.

I maintain that both birth plan advice and birth plans have political, material force. Even when plans are not "successful" for individual women's births, that political force resonates, affecting how women are treated and how they imagine, plan for, and experience childbirth. Online birth plan advice and templates, as well as physical (paper) birth plans, "make noise"—they create an "ideological disruption, in the mainstream discourses that dictate reality in both online and offline worlds" (Koerber, "Postmodernism" 236). This chapter uses invention (in the rhetorical sense of the creation and discovery of arguments) as a lens to show how online birth advice and birth plan templates convey and resist ideological meanings and commonplaces of childbirth and how these online tools serve, and also challenge, women's feminist rhetorical agency.

Women's invention of birth plans coincides with their attempts to invent themselves as patients, as birthing women, and as mothers in contemporary American society, often in ways at least somewhat resistant to dominant medical discourses and practices. The information available online (which is to say, information online circa 2005, in a largely Web 1.0 environment) that helped study participants invent their birth plans reveals a variety of complex and sometimes contradictory ways of understanding childbirth. This chapter's analysis of online birth plan advice and responses to a childbirth-writing survey also demonstrate that women's roles as consumers of health and medical information infuse their invention of their birth plans.

UNDERSTANDING BIRTH PLANS, FROM ORIGINS TO USES

Pinpointing the precise origins of the birth plan is difficult. An ngram[3] search for "birth plans" suggests a first published mention in 1945, but closer examination reveals that the earliest results refer not to the two-word phrase as it is used here but simply to the two words, often separated by punctuation, such as " . . . of Jones' *birth. Plans* for a formal . . ." (National Society 102; my emphasis). By the mid-1970s the phrase "birth plan" began to appear, though not as modern readers would understand it. Instead, "birth plans" in the 1970s referred to plans for birth control and fertility, that is, family planning, rather than plans for labor and delivery. Citations with this fertility control meaning cluster around policies in China, as in, for example, this 1976 explanation in the context of a cohort of workers: "All group birth plans are channeled upward where they are used to generate a master plan for the entire unit" (Chen and Zhen 96). But by the 1980s, birth plans as plans for labor and delivery started to appear.

Birth plans are now commonly associated with the Bradley Method, popularized by Robert A. Bradley, MD, author of *Husband-Coached Childbirth* (first published in 1965). However, Bradley's book does not itself mention birth plans, nor do such important works as Suzanne Arms's *Immaculate Deceptions* (1975), Richard Wertz and Dorothy Wertz's history of childbirth (1977), or William Arney's analysis of obstetric practices (1982). Jessica Mitford (1992) introduces the term as if it might not be familiar to readers, while Arms's second book (1996) describes a birth plan as "a list of the important features the parents want protected" (108). Arms goes on to assert that such plans demonstrate parents' instincts toward protection and "are the mark of a responsible parent, not a difficult patient" (108), suggesting that she anticipates that readers or at least physicians might have negative associations with the term. Postings on the thread "Birth Plans" on an obstetrical-gynecological Listserv (June 1997) indicate that some doctors then deemed birth plans "a West Coast thing"; many in other locations had not encountered them. Naomi Wolf (2001), like Mitford nearly a decade earlier, introduces the term without assuming readers' foreknowledge.

My survey respondents in 2005, however, all knew what a birth plan was, and half had written one. Some had learned about them from hospital information packets, others from "several books," and the rest online. Many had encountered the concept in multiple locations. One respondent with multiple children offered the explicit "I'm not sure if I heard of birth plans before the net." Combined, these responses suggest the Internet has played at least some role in birth plan proliferation. I suspect, too, that in the late 1980s and early 1990s, as women began to see the success of the second-wave women's movement and as women's empowerment in health care became visible through groups like the Boston Women's Health Collective, "writing back" to physicians and others in medical power became a tempting possibility to some women.

In *Infancy in America: An Encyclopedia*, Alice Sterling Honig, Hiram E. Fitzgerald, and Holly Brophy-Herb also assert that birth plans became popular in the 1980s; they attribute this to birth educators advocating for more parents to have choices in childbirth (87). Birth plans may have become more common in recent years because they are standard fare on the childbirth websites many women seek out when they become pregnant. An ngram search between 1940 and 2008 shows a graph with a fairly steady increase from 1980 on but with steeper, more significant increases in the late 1990s. Figure 2.1 provides a clear visual rendering of this trend.

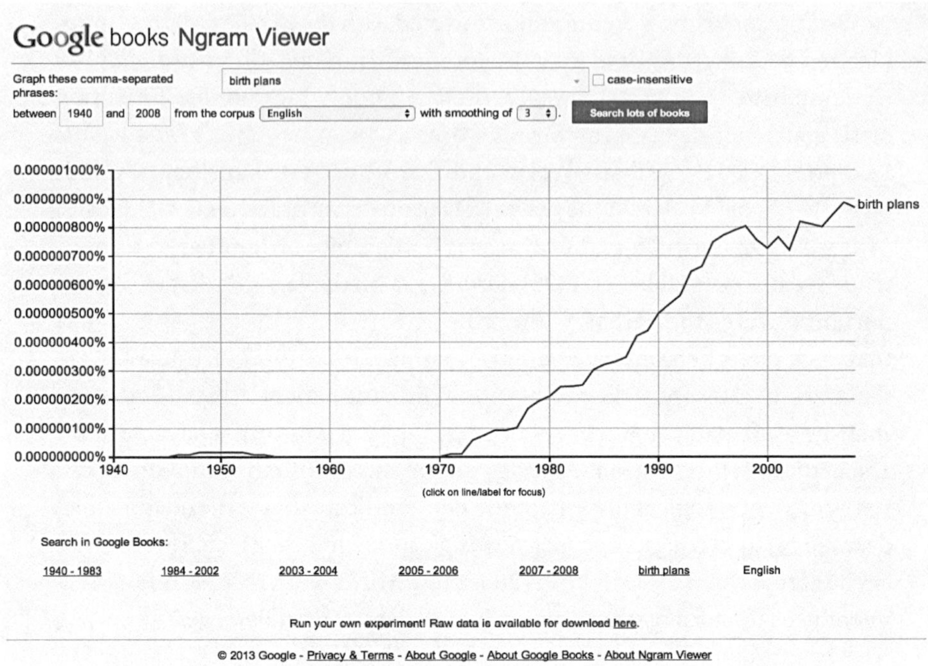

Figure 2.1. Ngram chart: frequency of "birth plans" appearing in books, 1940–2008

Even with the increasing popularity of birth plans, not all women write them, nor would it make sense for them to do so. "'[A] typical birth plan might say [a birthing woman] wants no IV's, no electronic fetal monitoring, would like to get up and walk around freely, be able to drink liquids, would prefer not to have an episiotomy, would like the baby with her as much as possible. Just simple things like that,'" explains nurse-midwife Mary Welcome (qtd. in Mitford 192). Women who would never question a typical American hospital birth[4]—who trust or assume that the doctor knows best—would be unlikely to write a birth plan asking for changes to the status quo. Because a primary aim of a typical birth plan is to prevent interventions perceived to lead to C-sections, those women requesting an elective Caesarean section would be also be unlikely to write birth plans.

From creation to implementation (or lack of implementation), the birth plan operates as a rare instance of patient-to-doctor written communication. Communication between doctors and patients is most often oral; a doctor takes notes and writes on a chart, but patients are rarely offered the chance to review those notes or even their own chart. When a doctor writes for a patient, this writing serves a transfer function; it possesses exchange value as a ticket for drugs or services from a specialized physician but does not convey information directed at the patient. The only writing that usually passes from a doctor to a patient, then, is a prescription or a referral, neither of which is written for the patient as its audience. This exchange function is underscored by doctors' use of abbreviations and Latinate terms and notoriously difficult-to-read handwriting.

As unlikely as doctors are to use writing to communicate with their patients, patients are, generally speaking, even more unlikely to provide their doctors with documents they have prepared. Birth plans created in anticipation of childbirth are a meaningful exception to this typical lack of written communication between patient and doctor. A birth plan is a form of written communication that seeks to reverse or at least interrupt the usual doctor-patient hierarchy (see Paget and DeVault on medical hierarchies and miscommunications that result). Women who write birth plans attempt to delimit and control the doctor's (and other staff members') actions.

My research suggests that women who investigate birth online and write birth plans absorb beliefs and values not only from medical information but also from outside medical ways of knowing. These range from person to person and birth plan to birth plan, but they include attempts to apply home-birth norms to hospital births, a rhetorical challenge with mixed results. For example, a birth plan might indicate that the birthing woman would like to have a medication-free labor, much like at a home birth, a fundamental element of which is a labor without pain medications. Women planning to birth without medications, whether at home or in a hospital, do expect pain (although a small percentage of women do not experience labor as painful), viewing pain as a bodily signal and an expected component of the event rather than as a symptom to be treated. This viewpoint appears explicitly in some birth plans, with requests like that in one survey respondent's birth plan: "Please do not offer me pain medication . . . [instead] please offer encouragement . . . or remind me of nonmedical choices such as changing positions." Such requests suggest attempts to borrow pain management strategies from home-birth situations and apply them to hospital situations; in a hospital environment, pain is typically responded to with medication.

Women I surveyed who wrote birth plans consistently described desires to avoid pain medications, a request of a piece with an overall attempt to demedicalize their childbirth experiences even while giving birth in medical institutions. Their reasons for writing birth plans suggest an understanding that pain medications are a common feature of contemporary hospital childbirth.[5] Sarah explained that she "wanted . . . as little pressure as possible from the doctors/nurses to have an epidural"; Kristy was "hoping that I wouldn't use any pain medication"; Marie "mainly saw it as a way to keep doctors and nurses from offering me pain medication and other (what I consider unnecessary) interventions." Cynthia brought a more global and forceful description, explaining that she wrote a birth plan "to let the nurses know not to mess with me and I mean what I say."

Lauren, who "had a bad experience with an epidural the first time," wrote a birth plan because she "wanted to have a natural birth the second time," thus contrasting birth plans with epidurals. She went on to explain that she also had a birth plan for her first birth but that "my doctor pretty much ignored it. The second time (different doctor) they were very agreeable to the birth plan and let me direct what I wanted, as long as it was medically safe." Lauren's experience of physicians and nurses paying more heed to the requests of a woman who has already given birth than to a primipara (woman giving birth for the first time) is a common refrain in childbirth narratives, suggesting that hospital attendants grant a certain deference to women's individual, experiential knowledge of childbirth.

On the other end of the spectrum, Julie, who did not write a birth plan, explained that choice this way: "I knew I wanted an epidural, so there was no way I was going to be one of those crazy women to do natural childbirth." Julie explicitly linked birth plans with "natural childbirth" (and natural childbirth with "crazy"!). Megan, too, set up a contrast between a birth plan and a desire for medication: "nope i did not have one! I only knew i wanted an epidural! that was it!" For these women, birth plans represented a way to avoid medications. These responses suggest that the writing of a birth plan was conflated with a desire for what they perceived to be a natural birth.

Women writing birth plans seem to rely both on their own ways of knowing and on their imagined or storied knowledges of others. Birth plans seem to simultaneously arise from and confront, or resist, educational as opposed to experiential knowledge. Women writing birth plans research and write as consumers, gathering educational knowledge about options (see Fletcher on childbirth consumption; Seigel, *Rhetoric of Pregnancy*, on pregnant women positioned as consumers; Shaw); they seem to be writing against a model of passive acceptance of medical interventions, acquiring multiple types of knowledges.

Birth plan writers in my study synthesized ideas from multiple sources, including pregnancy websites, birthing classes, online templates, and the ubiquitous childbirth preparation books, in addition to relatives, midwives, and physicians. One survey respondent, Sarah, wrote: "I hated most pregnancy books, especially *What to Expect When You're Expecting.* Found it really preachy and irritating and just generally awful. *The Girlfriends' Guide* was cute, wouldn't say it was so helpful though. I guess you have to read them, but they weren't so helpful, per se." Significant in Sarah's response is the somewhat offhand comment, "I guess you have to read them, but they weren't so helpful." While Sarah did not find the particular books she read helpful, she did feel required to read them. The "you" who *has* to read these books is a woman who aspires to be an educated consumer.

Sarah felt compelled to educate herself about pregnancy and childbirth; she consulted not only published texts but a variety of online resources, and she forged relationships in an online community of other pregnant women where she could learn from other women's bodily and educational knowledges. Other women in my study, too, wrote of extensive educational preparation. Kristy noted that she read "LOTS of books" and regularly visited a pregnancy website; Jessica "read a lot about twin delivery's thru twin books"; Anna "read anything [she] could find on the net" and "the 'What to expect . . .' book"; Karen described "tons of reading"; Marie "read a lot of books, talked to a lot of women, attended childbirth classes . . . [but] mainly followed the advice of women . . . who advocated natural childbirth." Several women remembered reading "lots of books"; some focused on particular types of births, such as PrettyMomma, who read "books about gentle home births." Nearly all attended a childbirth class (the only exceptions being women planning to birth at home outside the medical system).

Women's seeming compulsion for educational knowledge about childbirth (especially by middle- to upper-class, typically college-educated women like those who completed my survey) may result from their lack of experiential knowledge about childbirth. That absence of experience combined with the shift toward a consumer model of childbirth means that many women seek educational knowledge and can be bombarded with information. Much of that information is connected to what Amy Koerber describes as the "norm," that mothers are expected to be "obedient students who depend on expert advice from people who are often linked to consumerist, corporate culture either as part of the medical establishment or as producers and sellers of baby-oriented products" ("Postmodernism" 229).

And yet the myriad sources women encounter as they progress through pregnancy reflect multiple ideologies and stances that compete for prominence in influencing women's decisions about childbirth.

Women who write birth plans gather significant educational knowledge about childbirth. Interestingly, this educational knowledge often manifests itself in a desire to eschew, to some extent, scientific and technological knowledges (such as the educational knowledge that pain is to be treated with pain medication) and to instead rely on embodied, experiential knowledge (such as the notion that pain might be productive and handled without medication).[6] This blend of experiential and educational knowledge appears often. Marie's survey response illustrates this dual role: "Yes, I had a birth plan, I read about it in several books—particularly those which advocated a more natural approach to childbirth." Books (a form of educational knowledge) taught her to use writing (again, a form of educational knowledge) to prepare for a birth free from intervention (one relying explicitly on experiential knowledge in lieu of dominant educational knowledge while simultaneously in line with alternative educational knowledge).

The advice offered on childbirth and parenting websites, the ways birth plans are discussed in online birth narratives, and responses to my survey all suggest that many women write birth plans out of their desire for what they see as a "natural" birth process. Women surveyed wrote of wanting "as little pressure as possible" to have pain medication, "to let the nurses know not to mess with me," of wanting to "do natural" because of a dislike of needles. These documents, I argue, have a political force and demonstrate how women's rhetoric and ideologies codetermine their relationships with science, technology, and medicine.

Birth plans reflect societal concerns, but they also help shape societal concerns. In the next section I identify and examine how, in childbirth, rhetorical and political forces interact with temporal, physical, and spatial forces. I examine the material effects of medical and legal language on birthing bodies, looking at how language produces not only social realities, as Martin Nystrand and John Duffy suggest, but physical realities as well.

CONTROLLING BIRTH

While childbirth is a relatively unpredictable event, women have successfully controlled at least the circumstances of giving birth (in terms of location and attendants, for example) for centuries. That limited control over the event changed dramatically, however, in the early to mid-twentieth century when birth's location shifted from the home to the hospital (Leavitt, *Brought to Bed*). As hospital birth became the norm, women had less control over their births, not only in terms of attendants but in terms of technologies, medicines, and even freedom to move their bodies. By the 1980s, some women began writing birth plans in an effort to reclaim some control over birth without leaving the hospital. (There have also been women throughout this period who have given birth at home; legal and financial obstacles to this "option" are many and increasing, however. See Epstein; Hensley Owens, "Reviews and Reactions.") It may be that birth plans arose from a similar desire for reproductive control and women's health rights that led to the development of the Pill and to legal access to abortion. The level of control women have over birth control (conception) now, and childbirth itself historically, appears to exceed the level of control women in the early twenty-first century writing birth plans have over their hospital births in the United States.

Women expecting to predict and control labor and birth with anything like the accuracy with which they can prevent pregnancy are likely to be unpleasantly surprised (except, significantly, in the case of a planned C-section, which, whether planned for convenience or for medical reasons, does provide a relatively predictable, schedule-able birthing event—though still not one with controllable, guaranteed outcomes). Linda Layne, author of *Motherhood Lost*, argues that "childbirth educators who encourage pregnant couples to make a 'birth plan' obscure the extent to which pregnancy and birth are unpredictable, largely uncontrollable processes" (150). For Layne, who focuses on pregnancy loss, the issue of control is particularly poignant; she sees women who expect to control birth as unnecessarily traumatized by often inexplicable problems such as miscarriage and stillbirth. I agree with Layne that the birth plan as currently conceived can obscure the unpredictable nature of birth. Additionally, with a birth plan a woman seeks control over birth by asserting control over birth attendants' actions surrounding and responding to the birth—which many birth plan advice authors refer to as "interference" with birth. A birth plan's success, then, can be troubled as much by the "nature" of the birth itself as by the actions of birth attendants.

Birth attendants' actions are situated within the specific culture and rhetorical space of, typically, a hospital, where institutional policies, obstetric norms, and available technologies have tremendous rhetorical and material force. Recall that more than 99 percent of births take place in hospitals. The remaining births, fewer than 1 percent of all births, are spread between freestanding birth centers (0.2 percent of all births), home births (0.5 percent of all births), and clinics, doctor's offices, "other," and unspecified locations (Martin et al., "Birth: Final Data for 2006" 67). So for more than 99 percent of all American women's births, the hospital plays a significant role. And location is linked with control (or the lack thereof).

TIME: A RHETORICAL AND MATERIAL PLAYER IN CONTROLLING CHILDBIRTH

One of the most basic—and yet significant—obstetric norms and hospital policies has to do with the structuring of time. As Catherine writes in her birth story posted on *Plomp.com*, "In front of every bed there is a clock on the wall," a none-too-subtle indication that in a hospital setting, time matters. The concept of time may counter birth plan expectations because it is of primary significance in determining childbirth interventions. Jane Dwinell, labor and delivery nurse and author of *Birth Stories*, argues that childbirth is "no place for schedules and routines," a point that numerous midwifery texts and histories of birth support (see Arms; Arney; Davis-Floyd; Gaskin, *Spiritual Midwifery* and *Ina May's Guide*; Lang). In this vein, Beatrice, a woman experiencing an unassisted home birth, described time as standing "still—I had no idea what time it was, and I didn't care. I had no idea how often the contractions were coming—and I didn't care. I just let myself be swept away with them." By contrast, most birth plans and women's narrated experiences suggest that hospitals, in particular (as distinguished from less popular and less readily available location options, such as freestanding birth centers or home births like Beatrice's), often impose a schedule on birth.

The calculation and rigid scheduling of time are rhetorical obstacles a birth plan writer may unknowingly face. The midwifery model of childbirth sees the time of labor in terms of what rhetoricians call *kairos*, the ancient Greek term for "opportune time," or "opportunity," which has no English equivalent (Smith 47). *Kairos* carries connotations of "right timing"; Debra Hawhee explains that "*kairos* it not about duration but rather about a certain *kind* of time" (37). When seen as an intense experience of variable duration, as the midwifery model does, labor fits into this fluid notion of time, but when measured on a strict timetable, as hospital labors usually are, it is the Greeks' other conception of time, *chronos*, the kind of measured, linear temporality with which English speakers are quite familiar, that is valued.

An externally imposed *chronos*-based, rather than *kairos*-based, schedule actually begins long before birth, with the setting of a due date. Henci Goer, who identifies numerous disconnects between obstetrical research and obstetrical practices, finds that due dates are, more often than not, incorrectly calculated. She explains that "all clinical dating methods . . . have margins of error of more than two weeks" (180).[7] At first glance the discrepancy between due dates and birth dates may seem insignificant, especially since labor, as popularly understood, simply starts when it starts (a long-accepted *kairos*-based conception of time). And yet the rhetorical labeling of due dates has material effects, from shaping expectations of timing and disciplining the patient, in Foucauldian terms, to justifying a variety of interventions to start labor on a solely *chronos*-based schedule.

I should note that, as John E. Smith explains, *chronos* and *kairos*, while quite different, are also indivisible, which he explains with the example of wine making. Grapes must be harvested at the "right time," but this time is influenced by circumstances both chronological and *kairotic*. The wine maturation process, too, is tempered by both measurable time and a sense of quality—another "right time," or *kairos*. And yet in childbirth's *kairotic* moment, *chronos* overshadows *kairos*. For example, women considered overdue are perceived to be "high-risk" and are subsequently induced. Thus the issue of imposed scheduling can have significant effects on birth, both in terms of the woman's experience and the baby's health, because induction is not without attendant risks and correlated interventions.

Induction results in stronger contractions than natural labor produces; women thus endure more pain with less time to recover from each contraction, which increases the likelihood that they will want, need, or be offered analgesics and epidurals, which themselves affect labor, make birth plans obsolete, and can lead to what many women refer to as the "downward spiral" toward a C-section, perhaps following Naomi Wolf's phrasing. Numerous studies find that inductions lead to Cesarean sections (Goer 87–97). Beyond C-sections, "induction of labour . . . is associated with an increased incidence of foetal distress, uterine rupture, preterm infants and therefore more neonatal problems such as respiratory distress syndrome" (Oakley 25). Despite evidence suggesting problems with the practice, induction in American births seems to be increasingly common, with studies showing a rate of 9 percent for 1989, 18 percent for 1997 (Curtin and Park 4), and 21.2 percent for 2003–4 (Martin et al., "Births: Final Data for 2004" 3). Time constraints based on estimated due dates, then, easily supersede requests made in birth plans and can have direct and often negative effects on how labor progresses. It seems that whoever controls time controls birth.[8]

Because of miscalculated due dates—or rather, because of the rhetorical and material force that the very concept of due dates enacts in a corporate health care system—many women expecting to "allow nature to take its course" in labor, as many birth plan writers are, instead find themselves already subject to a schedule beyond their control, regardless of the careful wording of their birth plans. In this case, events are not simply out of anyone's control, as with a "natural" birth; the control in this case has shifted, both rhetorically and materially, to physicians and other birth attendants. Biomedicine has agency here; birthing women do not.

Induced births are not the only type of birth subject to fairly strict temporal schedules determined by the rhetorical space of the hospital. All hospital labors are subject to a schedule: doctors and nurses use an obstetric charting system that plots a woman's progress against a normalized temporal curve for labor, "a curve developed by Dr. Ernest Hill which defines on a graph how a labor should progress. . . . When a woman's labor is off the 'proper' curve, she is subjected to intervention in several possible forms" (Harrison 120–21). (It should be clear by now that any normalized notion of temporality is *chronos*-based.) While labors that move more quickly than the curve will simply result in babies being born, labors that move more slowly are defined as "prolonged." This definition, this rhetorical shaping of the situation, is not absolute, however. For example, Michelle Harrison also explains that the definition of "prolonged" changed significantly in the short space of fifteen years, from seventy-two hours in the mid-1960s to forty-eight hours in the 1970s to twelve to twenty-four hours by around 1980 (120). My interview with former obstetrician Judith Brysk confirms this shift, as do threads in a 1997 OB/GYN online discussion ("Birth Plans"). None suggest any change in women's labors, but the change in labeling, with a stronger emphasis on *chronos*-based time rather than on the *kairos*-based time historically applied to labor, has coincided with, and seems must have contributed to (along with other factors), the dramatic increase in C-sections over the last few decades.

Birth plans are often thwarted by a situation deemed dangerous (and sometimes actually dangerous), and time plays a significant role in the determinations of a situation's danger. The appropriate birthing time is to a certain extent a rhetorical construct, one situated in and affected by the times; as the discourse about time changes and becomes sedimented, so too do birth practices and understandings or perceptions of what is normal or safe versus abnormal or dangerous. Eviatar Zerubavel, a sociologist with a career-long interest in temporal relationships, writes in *Patterns of Time in Hospital Life* that the fact that hospital patients are referred to by units of time, such as "'a quickie,' 'a quick hit,' 'Mr. Quick,' or 'a quick buff' by house staff indicates that within the context of their daily work in the hospital, they often perceived of patients as temporal units of work" (91). Zerubavel was studying time patterns at hospitals in general, and my study does not examine precisely how doctors and nurses currently describe their patients; however, it does seem that doctors' and hospitals' uses and understandings of time have material effects on labor and thus produce material impediments to a birth plan.[9]

BIRTH PLANS CONTROL WHAT, EXACTLY?

> I really wanted my husband to cut the cord and I wanted to hold him right away and breastfeed to help expel the placenta, but none of that happened which was disapointing. Plus now my baby had a totally deformed head and a blister the size of the bubble in that game Trouble. Basically nothing went the way I'd planned. (Julie)

Women writing birth plans, as discussed, write in an explicit attempt to control the circumstances of their births. And yet that control might lie neither with the birthing woman nor with the birth plan, as was the case for Julie, whose three hours of pushing ended in vacuum extraction. Robbie Davis-Floyd, examining childbirth as an anthropological event, learned that couples "enter the hospital when labor begins expecting to retain control over the *birth*, although the method they are taught generally promises only that the laboring woman can retain control over her *behavior*" (184; emphasis in original). Davis-Floyd sees couples' belief in their control over the birth as misguided. While women and their partners write birth plans in which they make explicit choices about interventions they would choose and those they would not, usually emphasizing procedures they "hope to avoid," the ultimate control over what happens lies not with the couple or in that plan but in hospital procedures and the preferences of the birth attendants. Many birth attendants believe that their interventions are in the best interests of the patient, regardless of patient preference and despite medical research to the contrary, as Goer details in *Obstetric Myths versus Research Realities*. As Elizabeth Grosz explains, "Bodies are not inert; they function interactively and productively. They act and react. They generate what is new, surprising, unpredictable" (xi). Nowhere, it would seem, is this more true than in childbirth. The inability to predict and prescribe the actions and needs of the birthing body presents doctors and nurses with a ready explanation for deviations from birth plans, whether or not any given explanation is valid. Hospital staffs' beliefs about childbirth can (inadvertently or explicitly) undermine birth plans of women who seek natural (or as natural as possible) childbirth experiences.

Online birth narratives often suggest that expectant mothers believe in the power of the birth plan to deliver the type of birth they expect; when narratives mention birth plans, they are often described in terms of their not working or of their not being followed. Greta posted on *Childbirth.org*, for example, "I had a birth plan signed by my doctor. It didn't do me any good." Women I surveyed, too, lamented birth plans' not being followed. Shannon "expected that the nursing staff would respect my wishes . . . [but] [m]ost of the nurses couldn't conceive of me not wanting pain meds and weren't very helpful." Carla came to the conclusion that rather than setting expectations, "birth plans are more like wish lists!" Women writing birth plans may not be aware of the many medical and legal impediments to common requests.

Birth plans give couples what Naomi Wolf calls "a sense of consumer choice" (86). A *sense* of choice, however, may be all they offer. Michele, a woman who responded to my survey, corroborates Wolf's opinion. She looked at several birth plans online but created her own with input from her childbirth class instructor and her husband. She wrote: "I guess I mostly expected my birth plan to be a guide for my husband, so he could remind the staff of my wishes and expectations. My expectations were not met. After having given birth I see my birth plan as something for me to do *to feel like I had some control* over the situation, even though when the time came, I had zero control" (survey; my emphasis). For some women, this illusion of control prior to birth provides anticipatory comfort, which may be enough, but for others, like Michele, that prior illusion of control seems to heighten frustration when the birth experience differs significantly from the choices expressed in the plan.

Davis-Floyd explains how cultural forces inhibit the effectiveness of planned birth (although she doesn't use the term "birth plan," her focus on couple's expectations of control refers to a similar phenomenon):

> The expectation of the couple that they will be able to control the management of the birth often clashes with (1) the hidden cultural forces for socialization behind the application of obstetrical procedures; (2) the nature of the passive patient role that accompanies the definition of birth as a techno-medical event; (3) the fact that the couple is on hospital territory and is thereby placed at a tremendous interactional disadvantage; and (4) the fact that the couple would not *be* on hospital territory in the first place if they did not also share in the overall cultural definition of birth as a techno-medical event. (84–85)

Here Davis-Floyd neatly dissects the various ways in which expectant mothers and their partners are interpellated into the medical system, even though their educational knowledge about birth may have led them to believe in a different philosophy of birth from what Western medicine subscribes to. The sense of control birth plan writers develop might make them, in the end, less satisfied customers than if they hadn't expected control. Despite its implicit promises, the birth plan may be most effective as an educational tool for couples; through writing birth plans, women and partners learn, to a certain extent, what interventions might be suggested and what the range of women's experiences might be. The next chapter will explore the educational potential and rhetorical possibilities of the birth plan, such as women writing in order to control not only their attendants' actions but also their own and their partners'; here, though, I examine the various ways online advice shapes expectations and plans for birth.

ONLINE TEMPLATES AND BIRTH PLAN CONVENTIONS

Women do not create their birth plans in a vacuum. Rather, these documents are invented, in the rhetorical sense of arguments and ideas created, discovered, and/or shaped by one's situation and knowledges. Birth plans arise out of the information expectant mothers gather from other women, books, previous bodily experiences, birth attendants, and, increasingly, websites.

The sources women trust affect both the content and form of the birth plans that result. Some women rely on samples—birth plans that other women have written or that class instructors have created—while other women rely on what I am calling templates. Such templates offer document-production assistance and are prevalent on childbirth websites. They differ in presentation and content and go by various names: *Childbirth.org* offers an "Interactive Birth Plan"; *Birthplan.com* provides an "Online Birth Planner"; *iVillage* presents a "Personalized Birth Plan"; and *TheLaborofLove.com* includes both an instructive essay and a link to "Our Birth Plan." These birth plan templates operate as heuristics for childbirth. They help women invent their birth plans, showing women what they can and cannot do, what they may and may not ask for, what they should and should not hope for.

Environment:
Check as many as you would prefer.

- ☐ Dim Lights
- ☐ Peace and Quiet
- ☐ Music
- ☐ Wear my own clothes
- ☐ No students, residents, etc.
- ☐ Minimal vaginal exams *(Vaginal exams can actually cause problems such as infection and premature rupture of membranes.)*
- ☐ Other *(Please specify)*: ________

Mobility:
You may only select one.

- ○ Maintain mobility (Walking, rocking, up to bathroom, etc.)
- ○ Freedom to move in bed only (up to the bathroom)
- ○ Mobility not important (catheter, used with regular epidural)

Hydration:
You may choose a selection of these. For more information.

- ☐ No restrictions *(Eat & drink to your comfort)*
- ☐ Clear Fluids *(Water, Gatorade®, Jell-O®, etc.)*
- ☐ Ice Chips
- ☐ Heparin/Saline Lock *(Most hospitals require this as access to a vein should an emergency occur, it can also be used in place of an IV for administration of antibiotics for complications such as MVP or Beta Strep.)*
- ☐ IV *(You will have to have this if you are receiving medications.)*

Monitoring:
You may choose intermittent *or* continuous monitoring. For more information.

Intermittent Monitoring (ACOG Standards)

- ○ Fetoscope (Special stethoscope for pregnant moms.)
- ○ Doppler
- ○ External Electronic Monitor

Figure 2.2. Interactive birth plan template at *Childbirth.org. Courtesy of Robin Elise Weiss, MPH,* Robineliseweiss.com

It might help, at this point, to get a sense of what these templates look like, how they are organized, and what types of information are included. Figure 2.2, a screenshot of the first section of *Childbirth.org*'s birth plan template, shows what women see as they begin making choices. Various options are laid out in checklist format. Certain sections are text boxes, allowing women to write in their preferences, but the majority of this template is prewritten and would result in a bullet-point-style document, including only those options women checked off. Figure 2.3 shows a sample birth plan created using that template; in this sample we see how various categories (environment, mobility, hydration, and so on) from the template are collapsed into the single category "First Stage (Labor)." The template explicitly labels different types of data, allowing women to think through each possibility, but the birth plan itself is streamlined.

Birth plan templates are generally arranged in the usual order of birth: they start with the first stage of labor, offering options for mobility, position, environment, refreshment, and pain management. Many templates, in addition to providing some explanation of various choices listed, also provide

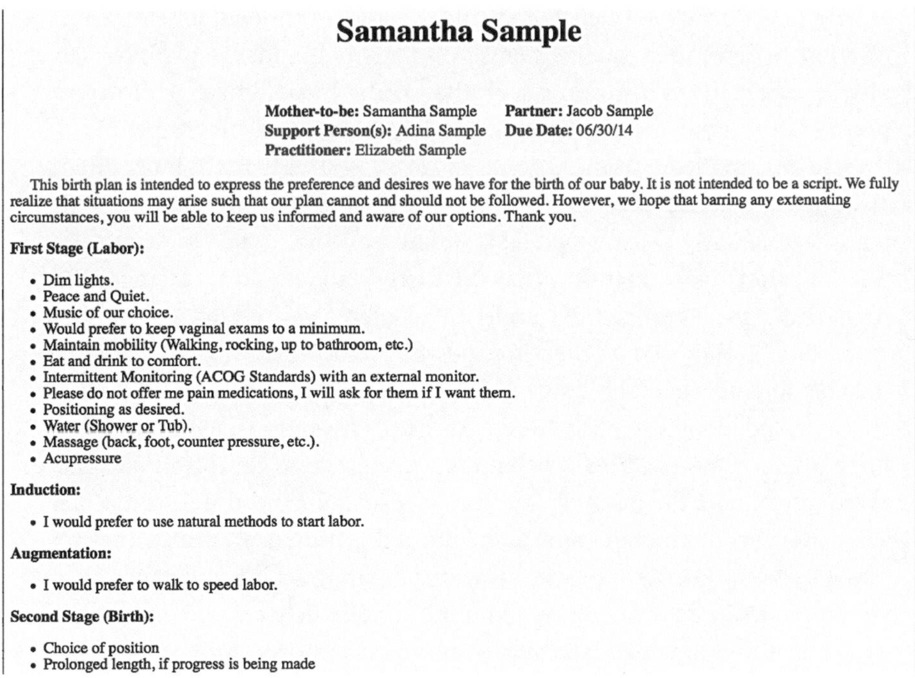

Samantha Sample

Mother-to-be: Samantha Sample **Partner:** Jacob Sample
Support Person(s): Adina Sample **Due Date:** 06/30/14
Practitioner: Elizabeth Sample

This birth plan is intended to express the preference and desires we have for the birth of our baby. It is not intended to be a script. We fully realize that situations may arise such that our plan cannot and should not be followed. However, we hope that barring any extenuating circumstances, you will be able to keep us informed and aware of our options. Thank you.

First Stage (Labor):

- Dim lights.
- Peace and Quiet.
- Music of our choice.
- Would prefer to keep vaginal exams to a minimum.
- Maintain mobility (Walking, rocking, up to bathroom, etc.)
- Eat and drink to comfort.
- Intermittent Monitoring (ACOG Standards) with an external monitor.
- Please do not offer me pain medications, I will ask for them if I want them.
- Positioning as desired.
- Water (Shower or Tub).
- Massage (back, foot, counter pressure, etc.).
- Acupressure

Induction:

- I would prefer to use natural methods to start labor.

Augmentation:

- I would prefer to walk to speed labor.

Second Stage (Birth):

- Choice of position
- Prolonged length, if progress is being made

Figure 2.3. Samantha Sample's birth plan (result from *Childbirth.org* template). *Courtesy of Robin Elise Weiss, MPH,* Robineliseweiss.com

hyperlinks to further information on options like walking epidurals, Pitocin, and nipple stimulation.[10] Templates then move on to the second stage, pushing. In this section templates may offer choices for delivery position, catheterization, and episiotomy versus tearing. After the second stage, many templates move directly to a baby care section, which might provide choices about cord cutting, bonding time, bottle- versus breast-feeding, and routine newborn procedures, skipping the third stage of childbirth, during which women birth the placenta.

What is striking, considering the array of sources and options for birth plans, are the constructions and content that are so prevalent they become conventions of the genre. Amy Devitt says that a genre "reflects, constructs, and reinforces the values, epistemology, and power relationships of the group from which it developed and for which it functions" (64). The birth plan, which has multiple functions for childbearing women—functions that range from educational tool almost to a contract—is a genre filled with conventions that rely on particular understandings of childbirth, many of which are borrowed from midwifery.

In sample birth plans, birth plan advice, and the birth plans I examined, certain conventions surface. For example, it is conventional for women to be polite in order to ingratiate themselves to their attendants; plans tend to phrase expectations beginning with the words "I would like" or "I would prefer." The modal "would" increases the distance between writer and addressee, making requests more polite and less assertive than the more direct "I want" or a command-like "do" or "don't." It is conventional for birth plans to explicitly resist expected hospital "routines," such as electronic fetal monitoring; to mention that the birth plan should be disregarded if anything goes wrong; and to refer to problems vaguely, as "emergency situations," rather than to mention specific predicaments (such as not being able to detect a fetal heartbeat, for example). The birth plan of Beth, a survey respondent, exemplifies each of these conventions. Beth opens her birth plan by saying, "I realize that I am not a medi[c]al professional and nothing can take the place of your knowledge and expertise. If situations arise that this birth plan cannot be followed, I understand fully. If at all possible I would really appreciate your help with the following items." She goes on to make specific requests about the labor, delivery, and baby care. That a birth plan, which is supposed to be an idealized version of women's *individual* expectations, consists largely of generic conventions might suggest a certain appropriation of women's individual rhetorical power. It could also, however, be seen as an example of rhetoric's dependence upon shared understandings.

In her essay "Invention and Inventiveness," Yameng Liu writes that "a postmodern sensitivity to the power/discourse nexus has alerted us to the fact that rhetorically significant 'topics' or 'commonplaces' have to be *authorized* by dominant political, institutional, or cultural formations in order to function as such" (53). Liu's argument suggests that birth plan conventions, or common topics, must somehow be authorized or sponsored. Because women consistently resist the dominant discourse of hospital births in their birth plans, sponsorship of those conventions does not arise from that institution; however, if Liu is right, they do enjoy dominance in some cultural formation—an alternatively dominant discourse, in other words. In this case, that "cultural formation" could be described as the midwifery model of childbirth.

If the birth plan is a document that seeks to challenge norms, as I believe it does, it is simultaneously a document that reinforces other norms, highlighting the idea that the act of invention cannot "effect a clean break with what is conventional, ordinary, commonsensical, and traditional or . . . transcend our socio-ideological situatedness and cultural inheritances" (Liu 60). The midwifery model, a minimally interventionist method of dealing with childbirth and one that relies upon women's and midwives' experiential and bodily knowledges, holds a certain status alongside and against the obstetrical model, which privileges scientific and technological knowledges and enjoys mainstream dominance in our society. Mary Lay explains in *The Rhetoric of Midwifery* that midwifery's continued reliance upon "touch and intuition" over "drugs and invasive procedures" both helps to define it and contributes to repeated confrontations over time about the issue of whose birth knowledge is "authoritative," the proper jurisdictions for and interventions into birth, and "the differing values of abstract scientific theory, principles of anatomy and physiology, and women's experiential knowledge" (43–44). Had the midwifery model not maintained some connection with what women perceive to be "commonsensical" and "traditional," its concepts would not appear in birth plans.

ONLINE TEMPLATES AND BIRTH ADVICE IN CONFLICT

Women turning to the Internet for help in inventing their birth plans discover a wide range of birth advice, birth plan advice, and birth plan templates. And while this proliferation of information has benefits, its vastness and contradictions, explored below, make demands of women's literacies. Birth plan writers may encounter, for example, birth plan advice written for physicians[11] or for lawyers rather than for birthing women, or contradictory recommendations on the same page or on linked pages. This section explores those kinds of conflicts.

Websites providing birth information often link to external sites that offer advice about creating birth plans. *Childbirth.org*, for example, links to various sites to explain the birth plan concept. Some of these links focus on the birth plan as a document *for women*, information I parse below. One, however, sends readers to a Louisiana State University Law Center page that describes birth plans in legal terms as a document for physicians ("Purpose"). The lawyer's advice, aimed directly at doctors rather than at birthing mothers, seems incongruous on this website for expectant mothers but is offered without explanation. This publicly available description reveals a legal, rather than prescriptive or communicative, purpose for the birth plan. The birth plan as conceived by the lawyer serves no empowering purpose. The site explains, "Physicians delivering babies should use birth plans to reduce conflicts and misunderstandings surrounding the delivery. Avoiding such conflicts can reduce the likelihood of litigation and improve the quality of medical care" ("Purpose"). The focus, then, is plainly on reducing lawsuits.

The birth plan invoked by this legal advice is not a document created by a woman to share her desires with her doctor; it is a document that doctors "should use." Although language about improving "the quality of medical care" is included, this is not presented as the main focus of the document. The document describes the three purposes of the birth plan:

> First, it structures the discussion between the physician and the patient. This ensures that all important issues are addressed with each patient. Second, it provides a framework for resolving inconsistencies between the patient's expectations and the risks of her particular pregnancy. Finally, it serves as documentation of the agreement between the physician and the patient. This will obviate questions about the information given the patient and any promises by the physician as to the management of the delivery. Legally most important, it will document the risks of pregnancy and the specific risks attendant on the delivery strategy chosen by the patient. This will not relieve the physician of liability for negligence. It will, however, bolster the physician's claim that certain injuries were foreseeable risks of pregnancy and not iatrogenic birth injuries. ("Purpose")

From the lawyer's perspective, the plan serves as documentation that patients were advised of their risks; any other benefits or purposes are incidental. Even the birth plan, then, ostensibly the woman's document, becomes instead a juridico-medical instrument.

By providing a format that "structures the discussion between the physician and the patient," the birth plan, from this point of view, privileges not a woman's choices but her doctor's desire to "structure" their conversation about the birth. If the physician is "structuring" this conversation (a structuring that may itself be constrained by hospital regulations or insurance policies), the woman's ability to convey her desires is always already limited. The hierarchical relationship of doctors and patients is only heightened if doctors are consciously structuring—arranging, organizing—this information exchange. Women who wish to challenge their doctors' choices, either before or after birth, not only must be willing and able to question or defy those in positions of authority over them but also must possess and activate critical literacies in order to unpack the underlying meanings of the language they, their doctor, or a lawyer includes in their birth plans.

Women seeking information as they write birth plans are not free of this obligation to weigh the value of conflicting advice when they click on other links from *Childbirth.org*, however. Another explanation of birth plans linked from *Childbirth.org* offers the following: "Birth plans are ideas and expectations that you have about the birth of your baby. . . . A lot of people misunderstand and assume you are writing orders for people to follow. Ah, if only labor would allow us to do this," author Robin Weiss seems to sigh. Weiss's explanation of a birth plan reveals both the "misunderstanding" that a birth plan is a document that binds the hospital to certain procedures and the belief that *labor itself* is in control of any deviations from a plan. As Wolf, Davis-Floyd, Harrison, and women's online birthing narratives (see chapters 4 and 5) make clear, deviations from birth plans often result from automatically applied hospital procedures or the preferences of birthing attendants rather than from the unique qualities of individual labor. One website offers this advice: "Remember that it helps to keep a birth plan short. Hospital staff can be notorious for not reading birth plans, so make sure your partner knows your wishes" (link from *About.pregnancy.com*). The birth plan, then, operates as a sort of genre of resistance, but one that may require oral backup. (This connection between speech and writing is explored further in chapter 3.)

As women decide which aspects of birth to embrace or resist, they rely upon the experiences of others, and yet since experiences differ dramatically, this source is not free of conflicts, either. The collective experiential and educational knowledges of those who create templates or offer online advice for birth plans are transformed into a codified, individually tailored document. Online templates guide women toward particular birthing choices, choices that reflect the underlying ideologies of those who create the websites. Even templates that appear to offer a full array of objective options may subtly guide women toward particular choices and away from others. Templates can easily restrict choices by not including them at all; like a highway map that neglects to include a particular road with the effect of keeping many people from driving on it, a template with missing items could keep women from considering the full spectrum of possibilities.

None of the birth plans or templates I examined, for example, makes any specific mention of stillbirth or miscarriage. Because a miscarriage is a real possibility for all pregnancies, and because a miscarriage handled in the hospital could be eerily similar to a live birth in terms of interventions—as Leslie Reagan points out, "the equipment used during pregnancy and delivery is also used during miscarriage" (357)—it might make sense to include wishes about such equipment in a birth plan. By avoiding the issue altogether, templates may unwittingly contribute to what Linda Layne describes as the alienation women feel—from societal expectations as well as from feminist ideals—when a pregnancy ends without producing a live child.[12]

Templates seem to fall into two categories: either they appear straightforward, presenting from what purports to be an objective perspective, or they explicitly advocate or seem to embrace a particular ideological stance. Upon close examination of the rhetorical choices of the template authors, however, readers will discover that ideological stances in templates are always present and not necessarily consistent. An ideological stance is sometimes compromised by contradictory statements. To illustrate, I quote from the sample "birth philosophy" from *Childbirth.org*'s template (a site that claims on its home page that "Birth is a natural process, not a medical procedure"):

> This birth plan is intended to express the preference and desire we have for the birth of our baby. It is not intended to be a script. We fully realize that situations may arise such that our plan cannot and should not be followed. However, we hope that barring any extenuating circumstances, you will be able to keep us informed and aware of our options. Thank you.

A cursory analysis of this "birth philosophy" reveals that while the first sentence is clear and logical and fits with the professed goal of a birth plan, most of the rest could be seen to undermine it. The second sentence begins already to infuse the "philosophy" with doubt—although no birth, surely, can be scripted, it seems unnecessary to mention this in one's birthing philosophy unless one is already resigned to its being, if not ignored, not followed. The third sentence serves more as a waiving of any rights—again, like a juridico-medical instrument—to have the plan followed than a statement of philosophy about birth; although, again, it makes sense not to impose a specific logic on any birth, by including this generic acceptance of "situations" that may "arise" (and with no mention of their occurring naturally or as a result of interventions, desired or otherwise), couples may, even in creating the birth plan, already be losing any physical or rhetorical claim over their birth. Birth plan authors are in a difficult rhetorical position, though, so such vagueness and acceptance may result from their attempt to create a reasonable, persuasive ethos.

The final sentence is the most counterintuitive, however, even taking rhetorical positioning into consideration. It does not, as one might expect, say that "barring any extenuating circumstances," this plan or our wishes should be followed. Instead, it says "barring any extenuating circumstances" (a phrase open to broad interpretation), "we hope . . . you will be able to keep us informed and aware of our options." The birth philosophy culminates not with a request that the attendants respect the desires of the couple or obtain their informed *consent* but with a request simply to keep them informed: thus, even as the plan professes to offer a woman or couple a sense of control over the birthing process, of which consent would be a small piece, the language included here gives up any claim to such control. The rhetoric of the sample birth plan, although overtly attempting to empower women and their partners, simultaneously and covertly undermines that power. The site suggests that the space is for "you to write your birth philosophy or whatever you want" and asserts that the example "can be erased and written over, used, or left blank," and yet the language of the example complicates women's invention processes and delimits their expectations.

Beyond complex issues like conflicting ideological stances or a seeming overabundance of information in online birth advice, women writing birth plans also encounter inventional difficulties because of information gaps. A key aspect of childbirth that many templates do not address is the third stage of labor—a stage many women don't even know about until they are pregnant. This stage is not typically depicted in movies or on television, unlike breaking water, contractions, and delivery of the baby. While some cultures place great value on placental tissue, like the Hmong, who bury the placenta after birth and expect it to serve as a protective jacket for the later journey to the afterlife,[13] Americans tend to see the placenta as bodily waste, which could partly explain popular culture's reluctance to display its delivery.

Procedures during the third stage can be controversial: some practitioners manually remove the placenta by tugging on the umbilical cord; other practitioners believe that the woman's body should expel the placenta without intervention; still others administer a routine shot of Pitocin to aid the expulsion. Each option has its advantages and drawbacks, and knowing about these options is important for women writing birth plans. As Liu suggests, we cannot invent out of whole cloth. While rhetorical invention has been conflated with both creation and discovery (problematic conflations, both, Liu points out), with birth plan invention, women need to discover the options available, not only to write the most effective plan in terms of their preferences but also because this stage is the most dangerous to women; the hemorrhaging that can occur in this stage can be life-threatening.

Birthplan.com is one of the few websites that offers options for the third stage of labor.[14] The template presents such options as "I do not want a routine injection of Pitocin after the delivery" and "I would like to hold the baby while I deliver the placenta" ("Online Birth Planner"). These options are embedded, however, within various requests for the baby, under the label "IMMEDIATELY AFTER DELIVERY" (emphasis in original), which suggests a certain problematic conflation of the two now-separate people being treated, and may interfere with women's ability to invent birth plans that take themselves and their babies into full consideration. Women relying solely on a single online template, then, might encounter rhetorical problems with significant material consequences. This issue, while particular to birthing women, illustrates the larger issue of people needing to learn how to evaluate online (and other) resources as life lessons for personal, health, and medical uses, not only for academic research purposes.[15]

All of the women I surveyed who had written birth plans used more than one resource—both online and offline—as a guide for their own plans. And even women using the web exclusively, seeking what Judy Segal calls "Internet health" information, are likely to consult more than one birth plan template, because multiple templates are linked even from single web pages, and to mix these models with advice from various sources as they create their own birth plans. Because women access various viewpoints, omissions and biases of particular sites may be less likely to inhibit the birth plan invention than if a given site were the sole source of information. Birth plans, which speak women's individual desires during labor, can also speak as a chorus comprising template authors and everyone else consulted in the writing.

The birth plan can resemble the patchwork that composition students often produce when first learning how to use and cite sources, or the boilerplate-style documents common in the business and legal worlds, where unique phrasing is less important than the sense a document conveys. While the documents are individually tailored, much of the organization and wording is often borrowed, which perhaps reflects pregnant women's necessarily limited time to acquire birth knowledge. The invention process, then, is not that of creating preferences from scratch; rather, women discover the possibilities and adapt their rhetoric to maximize their chances of achieving the birth they want.

One website, *TheLaborofLove.com*, provides women with a sociologist's detailed essay on birth plans; a link to a template is offered only at the end of this essay. This strategy makes it difficult for a woman at this site to simply use the template; first she must at least scroll through, if not carefully read, Amy Scott's "Eyes-Open Childbirth: Writing a Meaningful Plan for a Gentle Birth." The essay, like the templates on other sites, serves as a heuristic for creating a birth plan. Scott describes birth as

> paradoxical: a very predictable yet unpredictable human passage. On the one hand, almost without fail the vast majority of human females spontaneously begin labor, progress through increasingly intense stages of labor, feel like pushing, and give birth, at approximately 40 weeks after conception. On the other hand, reliably predicting birth in any greater detail than this is basically impossible. We cannot know the day or week labor will begin, how long it will last, exactly how it will feel, how we will react, or the health and sizes of our babies. What we can do, however, is educate ourselves about the vast array of possibilities and learn which are more likely to occur. We can decide what is ideal and what we will strive for, what are the means to creating the most conducive environment for such a birth, and which people can best help us to attain those birth arrangements.

Scott explicitly points to the birth plan as a tool of self-education rather than as a way to guarantee a particular outcome. While all templates do encourage women to learn about various birthing options, through offering sidebars of information or hyperlinks to more details, Scott's essay overtly recommends that women research fully and think deeply about what they want and can handle during their childbirth experience.

Scott suggests that women write narrative-style birth plans, rather than rely on what her birth attendant sources see as old-fashioned checklist-style birth plans. The differences between this site and others that offer checklist-style birth plans, then, seem readily apparent. Scott's position on birth plan styles may reflect the philosophy of *TheLaborofLove.com* in general, but this philosophy appears inconsistent among the linked pages. Scott's article gives nine pages of advice with no mention of relying on a template to accomplish this writing task, but then a link at the end of her article brings the reader to "Our Birth Plan," a template housed at *Mjbovo.com* (Fig. 2.4).

This template, the first of two linked from Scott's article, is particularly interesting because its options consistently contradict Scott's advice. The most glaring contradiction is that this template, which offers options for "what I would like to have during labor,"[16] results in a very short checklist with no space for narration at all. The phrasing tends to be in the form of short commands—"no routine IV's," "to NOT have . . ."—as opposed to the

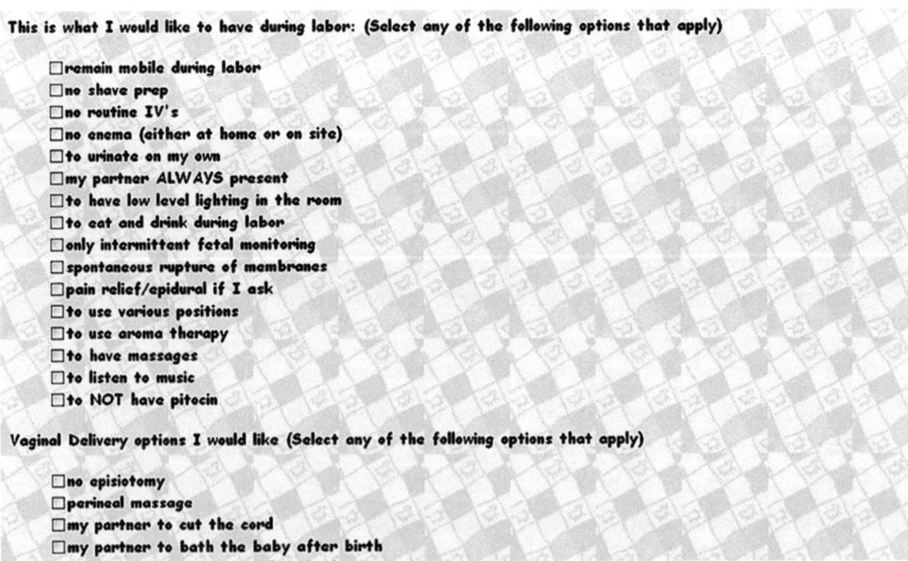

This is what I would like to have during labor: (Select any of the following options that apply)

- ☐remain mobile during labor
- ☐no shave prep
- ☐no routine IV's
- ☐no enema (either at home or on site)
- ☐to urinate on my own
- ☐my partner ALWAYS present
- ☐to have low level lighting in the room
- ☐to eat and drink during labor
- ☐only intermittent fetal monitoring
- ☐spontaneous rupture of membranes
- ☐pain relief/epidural if I ask
- ☐to use various positions
- ☐to use aroma therapy
- ☐to have massages
- ☐to listen to music
- ☐to NOT have pitocin

Vaginal Delivery options I would like (Select any of the following options that apply)

- ☐no episiotomy
- ☐perineal massage
- ☐my partner to cut the cord
- ☐my partner to bath the baby after birth

Figure 2.4. "Our birth plan." *Courtesy of Mary Jane Bovo, MD,* Mjbovo.com

"personal and thorough written description" Scott advises would be "helpful." She reveals that some birth practitioners believe "the short, concise style" to be outdated, quoting a doula who says, "'The old traditional bullet point birth plan is perhaps not the most effective thing'" (seemingly despite the relative ease of reading and absorbing such a format quickly).

Contradictions between the template and the essay extend beyond style to include content conundrums for birth plan writers. "No shave prep" and "no enema" are two of the first four options a woman may check; as Scott explains, though, "most hospitals no longer do routine enemas and pubic shaves; therefore, there is no need to write a request that it not be done. These sorts of written requests can be seen by some hospital personnel as insulting." A woman seeking to follow Scott's advice, then, might be confused by the format and content of the template she so easily reaches after reading the essay. Certainly the template's presence somewhat compromises Scott's rhetorical purpose and the ideology her rhetoric is intended to pass on to others, but this paradoxical juxtaposition also may serve to demonstrate to women that their birth planning process requires self-education that extends beyond the information available from a single online source.

Scott's essay encourages women to avoid the bullet-point style, treating that style as the standard from which women should now deviate. She asks women not to make requests to avoid procedures that are no longer routine in American hospitals, which demonstrates that birth plan conventions need to change as circumstances change. The essay and template, working together and against one another as they do on this site, may encourage women to seek other options beyond those listed on a template. Women following Scott's advice would pay attention to the *kairotic* elements of inventing their birth plans by noting which conventions might be appropriate to their particular situations and times. A woman might be inspired, for example, to check with her expected birth place about what is routine at that particular location so her birth plan could request differences from that specific routine, rather than rely on what a template expects to be usual practice. She may discover that online information, which is so easy to acquire and seems so helpful, can, as in the case of this template, be outdated, reflecting practices and conventions of an already bygone era.

Birth plans represent a technological and ideological confrontation of wills, the wills of birthing women, dominant culture, and medical staff. The outcome of this confrontation is determined through rhetorical strategy and rhetorical space. Birth plans are invented from a variety of sources whose commonplaces and ideologies are not always compatible with the commonplaces and ideologies in the rhetorical space—or rhetorical time—of the hospital. Birth plans signify differently for different constituencies (for example, birthing women, birth attendants, and attorneys). Such differences in meaning materially affect whether birth plans are implemented or ignored and how childbirth is experienced, shared, and remembered.

This chapter's examination of birth plan advice and templates reveals that the information provided within and linked from them is not of a piece but instead is often a contradictory palimpsest of ideas. Women writing birth plans must—and often do—sort a cacophony of often contradictory information out for themselves: they combine online research; conversations with attendants, partners, and trusted friends; and their own felt senses to create their birth plans, to begin to invent their births and assert rhetorical agency over them. Women's birth plan research and invention processes expose them to conflicting political, ideological, and consumer-oriented understandings of childbirth, gender roles, and medical hierarchies. This exposure has the potential to expand their epistemologies as individuals and, to invoke Koerber once more, to "make noise," disrupting the ideological dominance of a single way of knowing.

Women's carefully researched and invented birth plans often do not result in the births they planned. The rhetorical agency asserted in the birth plans does not uniformly result in material power. The next chapter analyzes individual women's birth plans obtained through my study and tells the story of those women's perceptions of those births; it extends the arguments begun here about the rhetorical complexity of childbirth and birth plans to explore the ways technologies and hospitals can silence birthing women while also explicating particular women's attempts to harness birth plans as tools of both resistance and self-education. It attends to how women use writing to confront the rhetorical disability inherent in many hospital birthing situations and asserts additional rhetorical possibilities of the birth plan.

CHAPTER THREE

CONFRONTiNG BiRTH

Rhetorical Disability and Five Women's Birth Plans

In her analysis of a do-not-resuscitate form (DNR), Lisa Keränen unveils the rhetorical shaping of end-of-life discourse, charting how institutional discourse guides families to make choices. Keränen writes that "the days leading up to death are marked by profound deliberations in which incompatible discourses converge around patients perched on the brink of being" (179). In childbirth, too, a different but no less profound event, women and unborn babies are each also perched on their own "brink of being." Childbirth, like death, was once a matter of the home but is now in the United States most often a hospital event rife with technological intervention, institutional imperative, and litigation potential. Also like death, childbirth is now often accompanied by written patient requests.[1] Like the DNRs and living wills that rhetorically shape (or attempt to shape, as Keränen shows) end-of-life decision making, birth plans, as described in chapter 2, rhetorically shape (or attempt to shape) decision making in childbirth.

This chapter extends the book's argument that regardless of the success of a birth plan, women who choose to write birth plans are asserting feminist rhetorical agency. Further, this chapter demonstrates that women write in part to combat a perception that agency will otherwise be absent in hospital childbirth. This chapter relies on and analyzes the five birth plans I obtained through my survey.[2] These five birth plans illustrate a variety of subject positions and orientations to technologies, physicians, and others who determine the applications of and interpret the signs of those technologies. The plans reveal the rhetorical challenges birth plan writers face in asserting their authority in the rhetorical space of the hospital.

While the rhetoric of the birth plan is often both carefully constructed and complex, birth plans do not seem to alter the power structures of birth or affect the application of technologies in the ways women might expect or hope. This study reveals, then, a seeming failure of rhetorical agency. At the same time, the study suggests that the process of writing a birth plan—an educational research and writing exercise—can nonetheless empower women.

I argue that a shift from relying on a birthing woman's bodily authority to relying on technological authority (outputs from monitors, for example) contributes to the perception or reality that she cannot communicate. Using a phrase introduced by Catherine Prendergast, who applies it in the context of mental illness episodes, I argue that women who write birth plans expect to be "rhetorically disabled" during childbirth. Birthing women are, or are positioned as, rhetorically disabled because they are experiencing pain; their temporary physical disability, along with other aspects of hospital birth, bring attendant rhetorical constrictions. "Rhetorical disability," here, refers to birthing women's (perceived) inability to communicate effectively due to pain, medication, an impaired mental state, and/or an imbalance of power between themselves and their attendants or between their own bodily authority and technology's authority. I contend that by writing a birth plan, a woman anticipates her own rhetorical disability, her temporary inability to speak for herself. Her writing is expected to stand in for her voice.

PERSPECTIVES ON BIRTH PLANS

Women who write birth plans for hospital births anticipate that they will help them control their birth, most often to avoid interventions (such as induction of labor, pain medication, epidurals, episiotomies) that are perceived to lead first to more interventions and then to C-sections. While women may write birth plans and expect to control their births, physicians, too, see birth as something that can—and indeed must—be controlled, both because of their training and because of fear of lawsuits. Medical malpractice suits are nearly always brought against obstetricians for *not* employing technological interventions when they could have, most often for not performing C-sections (Ecker and Frigoletto 888). Physicians' fear of litigation and consequent reliance upon technologies may be a significant impediment to a birth plan's implementation.

Physicians' attitudes toward birth plans range greatly—and may be changing. Birth plans were not immediately accepted by medical personnel, as the experience of Michelle Harrison, an obstetrics and gynecology resident in the 1980s, illustrates. Harrison describes seeing a fellow doctor storm out of a delivery room, yelling,

> "I hate patients like that! I can't stand taking care of them!"
>
> "What's up? Who is she?" I asked.
>
> "It's one of those couples who obtained signed agreements in advance stating exactly what they want and don't want. Her husband is hovering over her and won't let me touch her." . . . I was able to run some interference for the couple, especially in their not wanting an episiotomy. (176)

Harrison's willingness as a physician to enable the couple to avoid certain unwanted (and, based on the outcome, unneeded) procedures was unheard of among the doctors she worked with in the 1980s. A 1997 obstetric-gynecological email discussion reveals reactions ranging from supportive of patients' wishes to offense at various requests to a deprecating, "sordid" glee when anything prevented a birth plan's implementation ("Birth Plans"). Scores of contemporary online birth stories suggest continued resistance among physicians and nurses,[3] while other online birth stories reveal physicians and nurses working with women to implement at least some elements of their birth plans. Birth plans seem to wield inconsistent rhetorical and political force.

TECHNOLOGICAL OVER BODILY AUTHORITY

As technological and scientific knowledges have increased dramatically over the last century, so too has Americans' faith in those knowledges, which are perceived as superior to bodily knowledge. (By "bodily knowledge" here I mean an intuitive, tacit understanding of what one's body is doing and can or must do, as distinguished from bodily information mediated by technologies. Mary M. Lay uses "embodied knowledge" similarly [31].) Increasing reliance upon technological and scientific knowledge has a negative correlation with reliance upon bodily knowledge, which becomes suspect, if not dismissible, when read through the lens of technological, scientific knowledge. It is through this lens that most women encounter pregnancy and childbirth: bodily signals are repeatedly subsumed to technological signals, from the discovery of pregnancy through delivery. Various scientific tests whose results require interpretations are performed on (and sometimes by) women. Because the course of hospital births tends to be determined more by technological than by bodily knowledge, technologies and those who control them perpetuate a particular kind of rhetorical activity while silencing another.

Technology can serve to silence women and to supplant, rather than supplement, bodily knowledge: This shift in the hierarchy of knowledges is one reason that some women have begun writing birth plans. Birth plan authors (re)educate themselves about birth using the technologies of writing and reading available to them, from the Internet to books to other women's birth plans. Through their research, many women come to believe in the potential of bodily knowledge, which leads them to try to resist childbirth as a technologically mediated event. Julia, one of my survey respondents, for example, describes herself as "an educated consumer, rather than someone who did whatever my dr thought was best. With education comes options. I do not think drs have time to educate each of their patients on all the options available and I don't think some drs care to do so b/c they like to be in control." For Julia, education meant taking some control for herself. Like many birth plan writers, she sought a delivery free of any technological interventions. (And unlike many birth plan writers, she succeeded.)

Hospital births are notoriously punctuated by various technological interventions, any one of which can lead to a "downward spiral" of multiple interventions that can result in an "emergency" C-section (see Wolf). Although women write birth plans to avoid these interventions, most of the women I surveyed and whose online birth narratives I read found their birth plans of little help. Naomi Wolf finds that birth plans are publicly laughed at by some nurses and that hospital protocols usually trump women's birth plan wishes (82).

Women who write birth plans do so in an attempt to prevent the seemingly inevitable transference of bodily authority to technologies and those who use/interpret them. But not all women birthing in hospitals seek to avoid technologies; many women expect technological birth assistance, often in the form of pharmacological pain relief. However, these women are far less likely than technology avoiders to write birth plans. For example, in response to the survey question "Did you have a birth plan?," Julie wrote, "I knew I wanted an epidural, so there was no way I was going to be one of those crazy women to do natural childbirth." For Julie, as for many women, birth plans are equated with natural childbirth. One implication here is that "natural childbirth" is, to women like Julie, an aberration. Another complementary implication, however, is that some women are less likely than others to be concerned about the potential for technologies to be rhetorically enabled when they themselves might not be. For some, a shift away from bodily and rhetorical authority during childbirth is not only expected but welcomed.

Women who write birth plans are using technologies of writing (including computers and online advice and templates) to confront technologies of birth. I show that these choices are rhetorical but that their effect is limited in the rhetorical space of the hospital.

FIVE WOMEN'S BIRTH PLANS

The five birth plans I analyze here illustrate how medical, legal, and narrative discursive styles converge in this birth advocacy genre. The women who wrote these plans relied upon various strategies to try to make their expectations understood. Characteristics of the five birth plans in this study are summarized in Table 3.1.

The majority of my survey respondents who wrote birth plans consulted online templates and advice. Other sources included their care providers and birthing classes. To prepare for my analysis of the birth plans, I examined the sources my respondents and I both had access to—online templates and birth advice sites—in order to become familiar with the features and content of birth plans that would result from those. To analyze the birth plans, I first looked for features that aligned with or deviated from what I had come to expect from online templates and advice.

Most online templates provide checklists and will produce simple bulleted lists. A request resulting from such a template might begin with the word "no" and follow with an intervention like "episiotomy" (see, for example, the "Interactive Birth Plan" at *Childbirth.org*). Competing but less prevalent online advice suggests that bulleted checklists are somewhat outdated (interesting, given the apparent youth of the genre itself) and encourages women to narrate requests instead (A. Scott). The birth plans in my archive reflect a range and mixture of these disparate generic styles; even birth plans influenced by online templates are personalized far beyond what simply filling out the online form would produce.

After determining how the styles and features of my five plans matched up with template-derived expectations, I generated conditional categories of features, such as politeness strategies, which recurred across the five plans, and others that were anomalous among the batch, such as legal language. I compared the birth plans with one another and with women's survey responses about their births and birth plans (and, where possible, their birth narratives).[4] Each round of comparison yielded more interesting nuances of features on which to focus.

Table 3.1. *Five Women's Birth Plans*

	Carolyn and Eric	RH and BH
Birth number	First	First
Birth location	Hospital	Hospital
Pronouns	"I"; "we"; "our"	"I"; "our"
Style	Nonnarrative bullet-point	Mixed: narrative and bullet-point
Excerpts demonstrating style	"• To breastfeed soon after delivery." ("WE WOULD PREFER" sets up the bulleted list.)	"As soon as our baby is delivered, please place him on my chest or abdomen . . . I would like to breastfeed him immediately."
Excerpts demonstrating politeness strategies	"WE WOULD PREFER a drug free delivery."	"If I ask for medical pain relief, please offer encouragement or remind me of non-medical choices."
Excerpts demonstrating appropriation of hospital "routlnes"	"WE WOULD PREFER to postpone 'routine' newborn procedures until we have had a chance to bond with our baby."	"Please, no routine preparation tasks (enema, shave, etc.) unless requested."
Excerpts demonstrating ethical appeals	"First—*Our number one goal is to have a healthy baby and a healthy mom!*" (their emphasis)	"I tend to tense up when I am around people with whom I am not intimately familiar. So, it would be favorable if my husband and I were alone as often as possible."

Julia and Greg	Beth	Karen and Sander
First	Second	Third
Birth center	Hospital	Home
"we"; "she"	"I"	"we"; "she"
Nonnarrative paragraphs	Mixed: narrative and bullet-point	Narrative paragraphs
"Breastfeeding will be attempted immediately following delivery."	"• I would like to hold the baby immediately after birth."	"Karen plans to breast-feed as soon as possible, and we would like our child to be checked out while he is lying on top of Karen."
"Please do not offer pain medications, we will ask for them if Julia wants them."	"I would like a drug-free delivery."	"We hope not to use the hospital at all, but if we need to transfer, we are looking forward to having a positive birthing experience with your assistance."
"Vitamin K shot is not to be administered routinely."	"In routine circumstance I would like all procedures explained to me before they are performed."	"Karen does not want to receive a routine episiotomy, she prefers to risk a natural tear."
"Mobility is important to us. Please keep vaginal exams to a minimum and only do intermittent monitoring, following ACOG standards, using a fetoscope."	"I would like to avoid tearing. I would rather have an episiotomy. I realize that this is often just a judgment call on the part of the physician, but I tore badly last time and I am scared of that happening again."	"We are Dutch people who . . . come from a country where home births are normal and hospital births have a minimum of interventions. We had our first two babies at home . . ."

The categories I share in Table 3.1 represent the features of the birth plans I argue serve rhetorical functions. (The table also includes information important to the context and some content of the birth plan, such as birth location and number of birth.) The wide range of features on display in this sample of five birth plans is suggestive of the importance of the genre of the birth plan for rhetorical scholars who seek to understand how everyday people use writing in and for their lives, or more particularly how people use writing to affect their medical encounters.

Beyond generic style and content, features on which I focus the analysis include pronouns, politeness strategies (such as indirect requests, use of modal constructions, and saying no to particular interventions without writing "no"), legalese, "routines" and other medical discourse, and ethical appeals. Each of these features is analyzed in its own section below.

Pronouns

Pronoun choice was one of the first features of the birth plans that stood out as I tried to understand not only the birth plans themselves but also women's processes of creating them. One might expect a woman's birth plan to use the singular first person pronoun "I" since, after all, the woman herself is giving birth. But the birth plans in my data set employ multiple different pronouns (see Table 3.1). The decision to write "I" or "we" may reflect a woman's expectations that birth is either something she does, hence "I," or something she and her husband do, in which case she would write "we." (And here I should note that every woman in my study was married to a man.) Four of the five birth plans mention husbands by name and employ plural pronouns at least part of the time.

Beth was the only one of the five to have a birth plan that exclusively uses the pronoun "I." Her choice may reflect the influence of the online templates she relied upon, each of which I examined as part of my study and all of which also use "I" exclusively. She, like the others, however, availed herself of sources beyond the online template archive. The decision to use particular pronouns may result from templates, advice, or embedded beliefs about birth, but it also may be a grammatical manifestation of women's desire to control birth.

Beth's birth plan is compelling for its consistent use of "I" and its insistent appeal to herself as an empowered agent. Despite Beth's obvious belief in her ability to control her birth—the plan indicates that she wants a drug-free delivery, to choose her delivery position, and to hold the baby immediately afterward—she nonetheless expects significant assistance from her birth attendants. Beth's plan is not exclusively noninterventionist; in fact, she *requests* certain interventions, in stark contrast to the other birth plans I examined through the survey and online. Significantly, she "would like to be offered an enema," "would like to be catheterized," and "would rather have an episiotomy" than a natural tear (although she wanted all involved to help prevent an episiotomy, too).

Beth's requests, then, directly contrast with the requests the other four birth plan authors make—Karen and Sander, for example, write, "Karen does not want to receive a routine episiotomy, she prefers to risk a natural tear." Beth's requests also contrast with the options presented in online templates, which offer suggestions such as "would prefer no catheter" and encourage avoiding enemas. Most such options in the templates I examined are phrased in the negative for medical procedures; there is no box to check for "I would like an enema, please." Beth, then, seems to be writing against a traditional birth plan in that she requests the very interventions others seek to avoid. Beth's plan highlights the way even birth plans based on online templates can nonetheless be individually authored—her requests are highly idiosyncratic compared to other birth plans and reflect her particular bodily, educational, and experiential knowledges.

Birth plans that employ the first person plural ("we," "our") also reflect particular knowledges, but the pronoun use can present the idea that birth is a family event, not solely that of the birthing woman. Through sentences like "We have prepared very well for the birth by following childbirth classes and reading a lot and we expect to be part of the decision making when interventions are needed" (Karen and Sander), women ensure that their husbands are seen as integral to their labor and delivery. (This may be an extension of the intriguing tendency of some couples to announce, "We're pregnant!") Women may grammatically include husbands or partners in their birth plans to inform or remind birth attendants that when/if the birthing woman herself is unable to communicate, her partner is authorized to speak for her, for them. Julia and Greg's plan, for instance, includes this request: "Please do not offer pain medications, we will ask for them if Julia wants them." The pronoun usage in this sentence suggests that the couple is open to Julia's desires changing in the moment and expects her wishes to be met, but that any specific requests on her part will come not only from her but from them. Through its collective pronoun use, this birth plan conveys the idea of a united front.

Beyond establishing a particular view of birth, "we" may suggest that both partners participated in writing the plan; however, of these five women, only Julia overtly described actually writing the birth plan together with her husband. Beth stated simply, "I wrote it by myself" (survey). Of the other sixteen women in my survey who wrote birth plans, eight describe writing them with some help from their husbands; five remember writing them alone; two are less explicit but exclusively use "I" when discussing their writing processes; and one cowrote with a midwife.

Women who use "we" in the birth plans they write alone may do so not only to announce to the hospital staff that their partners are to be involved but also to encourage their partners to participate. Using "we," then, may be a subtle rhetorical strategy aimed at someone other than the target audience for a birth plan. While pronoun use may suggest consideration of both expected and unexpected audiences, other features, such as politeness features, point to careful consideration of the expected audience of hospital birth attendants (physicians and nurses).

Politeness Strategies

Multiple politeness strategies appear in four of the five birth plans I examined. Even the fifth plan, which is distinctive instead for its tendency to use direct, command-like requests, uses words like "please," suggesting at least a limited sense of politeness. These opposing features reveal much about how women attempt to encourage or dictate birth attendants' actions.

Some may view "politeness" as a form of ingratiation, a problematic presumption of birth attendants'—particularly physicians'—superiority. I have come to see politeness strategies instead as a rhetorically savvy understanding that the power structure of the hospital strongly favors attendants over patients. It is perceived to be easier to get something by saying "pretty please" than by making demands, and a certain degree of subordination by patients fits with the cultural reverence shown to physicians in American society. Women seeking to reject pathological interpretations of childbirth—which many, if not all, birth plan writers are—need to connect with their audience somehow. Birth plan authors can cite educational knowledge, but medical staff may be dismissive of such claims.[5] Those who have given birth can cite that experience to assert a certain bodily authority. But a consistent rhetorical strategy in the birth plans I studied is to make exceedingly polite requests rather than commands or demands and to offer suggestions for the ideal situation (with the often explicit acknowledgment that no birth is likely to be an ideal situation).

Penelope Brown and Stephen C. Levinson's landmark text[6] in politeness theory, *Politeness: Some Universals in Language Use*, posits that politeness strategies are all about maintaining the "face" of both speaker and hearer.[7] Brown and Levinson describe "face" as "something that is emotionally invested, and that can be lost, maintained, or enhanced, and must be constantly attended to" (61). Further, they argue that people mobilize polite terms and constructions in order to save their own faces and those of the people they address. They split politeness into two basic categories: positive and negative. Positive politeness maintains the face of the addressee through friendly treatment and establishing shared desires and status, while negative politeness (which does not carry the negative implications one might expect) seeks to maintain the addressee's territorial claims and freedom of action through deference, formality, hedging, and distancing strategies (70). Negative politeness, which is expected in asymmetrical social relationships like those that birth plan writers have with medical staff, is fairly common in the birth plans I examine.

One rhetorical choice that distances the writer and audience is modal constructions. Auxiliary verbs such as "would" soften requests; such softening, according to Brown and Levinson, smooths the interaction, making it less likely that the addressee will feel impeded or coerced. Such constructions litter birth plans. Carolyn and Eric write a bullet-point-style plan, in which sentences are completed by a boldface "We would prefer" at the top of the page. RH opens her birth plan with a gracious "First of all, I want to thank everyone in advance . . ." before moving on to describe preferences like "it would be favorable if my husband and I were alone as often as possible." Beth uses the phrase "I would" fourteen times in her twenty-one-sentence birth plan. These modal constructions are less direct than statements like "I want" or "we desire." Such indirectness is a common element of polite discourse and in birth plans attempts to save the faces of medical staff.

Beyond employing modals, some birth plan writers further soften requests by tending to phrase them without saying "no," so a request for no drugs is written "I would like a drug-free delivery" (Beth) or "We would prefer a drug free delivery" (Carolyn and Eric). RH combines direct use of "no" with somewhat contradictory requests, both grammatically and in terms of content. She writes, "Please do not offer me pain medications, I will ask for them if I want them." In other words, she first asks not to be offered pain medications but lessens the negative impact of this direct request by saying she will ask for them if she wants them. The latter part of the sentence serves a face-saving function for medical staff trained to relieve pain through medical means.

Immediately after this fairly straightforward request, however, RH writes, "If I ask for medical pain relief, please offer encouragement (ex: 'but you're doing so well!') or remind me of non-medical choices such as changing positions." Here, RH's construction is somewhat convoluted. Although she maintains a basic level of politeness with constructions such as "please offer," she essentially asks her care providers to hear one request (for pharmacological pain assistance) and respond to another (for nonpharmacological pain assistance). This contingent request attends much less to face-saving, both because of what it asks and how it is asked; it also demonstrates RH's awareness that she may not be able to ask for what she wants at the moment of birth. The above examples, which attempt to achieve the same goal through different rhetorical means, are short. While indirect enough to be polite, even ingratiating, they are direct enough to be read quickly. Keeping a birth plan short shows a certain accommodation of attendants' time, a further indication of politeness and respect.

Legalese

Julia and Greg's birth plan provides a counterexample to the politeness principles demonstrated above in that it makes use of fewer indirect statements and has, in general, a significantly less polite tone. This difference in tone may result from their belief that the birth plan is an explicitly legal document, much like a DNR.[8] While they do use words like "please," Julia and Greg often phrase their comments fairly directly, using "we desire" to set up preferences. They also phrase certain statements in command form rather than as requests; for example, the plan ends with this ominous and legal-sounding statement: "This plan is to be altered only with the consent of Greg and/or Julia, unless there is a life-or-death emergency." Here the authors set up their plan as more of a contract than a list of preferences.

Julia and Greg also demonstrate their educational knowledge of childbirth by making requests that are simultaneously lessons: "Please allow the placenta to expel naturally. Do not pull on the cord or administer medication to speed this. The baby breastfeeding will help this." Although the paragraph opens with the word "please," there is little sense here of ingratiation or submission to medical authority. An imperative statement follows the initial request; "do not" appears instead of the "we would prefer to avoid" construction so common in the other birth plans and online templates.

Beyond this, the final sentence might offend birth attendants, who are rather likely to be aware that breast-feeding stimulates the uterus to contract. This plan does not apply negative politeness strategies: no effort is made to defer to and/or save the face of the addressee.

Unlike many birth plans, which simply include names of parents, caregivers, and sometimes the expected baby, Julia and Greg's plan, as well as RH and BH's, include spaces for the signatures of the woman, her husband, and the certified nurse midwife. The signatures attempt to confer a certain legal authority over the birth plan, perhaps expecting them to function like DNRs, which "only" become "a formal order for the chart when signed by a physician" (Keränen 186). Julia, who used a Bradley Method birth plan template and an online "interactive one" to customize the birth plan she wrote with her husband, believed that

> birth plans that are signed by your caregive[r] become an advanced directive for the hospital and are legally binding. This also confirms that your caregive[r] and you are thinking of the upcoming birth in the same manner. My first dr would not sign off on my birth plan. This was the deciding action for switching caregivers. I had inklings before but him disagreeing with my birthplan showed me that he and I were not compatible. (survey)

Julia's belief in the legal power of her birth plan to prescribe what would happen was somewhat misguided, but it certainly shaped her rhetoric.

Her comment also displays the usefulness of writing the birth plan, however, since through this compositional act, she gained particular knowledges and expectations with which she was unwilling to part. Julia's writing of a birth plan led to discussions with her doctor, which in turn led her to choose a new caregiver and birth location (perhaps significantly, she chose a certified nurse midwife and a birth center to replace an obstetrician and a hospital). Julia's experience highlights the material effects such writing can have; the stakes of such writing are formidable.

"Routines" and Other Medical Discourse

While Julia and Greg's birth plan contains the most explicitly legalistic language of those I had access to, other of its features are common among all of the birth plans, notably its use of the word "routines." In hospitals, "routine" is a term usually used by and in the interests of hospital staff, but in the birth plans the term is appropriated as a method of resistance.

Each plan refers to hospital "routines," though each does so in a slightly different way. Table 3.1 includes a sample of how each birth plan mentions what is routine in the hospital. For these women, hospital routines are treated as something to avoid or adapt. Carolyn and Eric, for example, prefer "to postpone 'routine' newborn procedures until we have had a chance to bond with our baby." They not only use the word "routine" in the birth plan but mark it with scare quotes. They use the word and the quotation marks together to preempt what they anticipate will be used as a rationale for unwanted separation. They seem to perceive "routine" to be a word that possesses significant rhetorical force in situations where a hospital's "routines" can easily trump a patient's desires or expectations.

The emphasis on routine reveals that these women and couples are quite knowledgeable about general birthing practices, a knowledge acquired through reading and classes. By highlighting the word "routine," Carolyn and Eric question the rationales behind routines; they seek to triumph over Carolyn's anticipated rhetorical disability in the face of these routines. The rhetorical tactic here is to take a term commonly used by medical professionals—one used to encourage compliance, to invoke unnamed authority—and bend it to the patient's will. The way birth plan authors use "routines" sparked my interest in other medical discourse the birth plans (re)appropriate.

Birth plan authors incorporate medical discourse—a possible display of educational knowledge—into their requests in varying degrees. Carolyn and Eric's request for "a chance to bond" is shared in spirit, though not in precise language choice, among all five birth plans. Julia and Greg and RH and BH use common medical parlance, asking for the baby to be placed "skin-to-skin." Karen and Sander rely on more colloquial phrasing; they would like the baby "on the mother's belly." Carolyn and Eric clarify they want the bonding to take place "on my [Carolyn's] chest," and Beth would like to "hold the baby immediately after birth." Western scientific research (as early as Klaus and Kennell, 1976) supports immediate skin-to-skin bonding for maternal-infant attachment and successful breast-feeding. Current research (Mizuno et al.) suggests that initial contact between baby and mother—for at least fifty minutes just after birth—causes the baby to better recognize the scent of its mother's milk and increases the extended success of breast-feeding. Such findings seem to be ignored, however, in determining the timetable for routine newborn procedures (such as weighing and applying eye ointment) in hospitals: "routine separation shortly after hospital birth is a uniquely Western cultural phenomenon that may be associated with harmful effects including discouragement of successful breastfeeding" (Anderson et al.). While birth plan authors may not be aware of the body of research supporting immediate breast-feeding, their requests signal recognition that many hospitals routinely disallow or (at least inadvertently) discourage immediate breast-feeding.

Birth plan authors, relying as they do on advice from multiple sources, often gain particular educational knowledges about medical, or scientific, discourse. Because the dominant vocabulary for birth in our society is medical, even those attempting to resist a medical definition of birth must rely to some extent on medical terminology, whether they understand it or not (on "resisters" appropriating dominant discourses, see Mentor 75). Some women may include such discourse in their birth plans simply because it is available on websites and templates, without a clear understanding of its meaning; others, however, possess significant knowledge about childbirth. Like Julia and Greg, who demonstrate their understanding of how breast-feeding can assist with delivery of the placenta, Karen and Sander display educational knowledge when they write, "We prefer you not to clamp the mother's side of the cord, to reduce the risk of Rh sensitization." Their tone is semi-instructive, though also politely phrased, their knowledge displayed but subverted; they briefly and gently narrate their request using medical terminology. Such medical discourse is threaded throughout all of the birth plans and templates I analyzed, including terms and phrases ranging from "catheterized" to "episiotomy" to "intermittent monitoring with a fetoscope or Doppler."

When women and couples incorporate medical discourse into their personal birth plans, they seem to do so in an effort to convince birth attendants that although their requests are personal, they also are grounded in educational knowledge. Birth plans, while necessarily personal, also aspire to be professional in that they adopt professional discourse to make demands and requests. Couples may try to demonstrate through medical language that their understanding of birth procedures is scientifically and educationally derived and that their particular desires stem from knowledges developed through research and careful consideration rather than on a whim. They draw on various discursive models, from midwifery and from medicine, as appropriate, and often together. These discursive choices, however, may alienate rather than persuade.

Former obstetrician Judith Brysk noted that when she would ask women why they wrote a birth plan, some would respond, "The online site said we need[ed] to do this." Partly because of responses like that, Brysk felt that women rarely "knew what those decisions [birth plan requests] were about." She was generally able, in pre-birth discussions with women about their plans, to convince them to focus on trusting her as a physician rather than trust what she saw as their limited knowledge about childbirth. Brysk constructed patients as relatively ignorant about childbirth. For her, medical training and experience with hundreds of deliveries easily trump educational knowledge on display in a birth plan. She was willing to go along with birth plans as long as everything was "going great," but she felt the plans offered women a false sense of security and caused disappointment. Brysk, then, was one obstetrician on whom women's rhetorical strategy of harnessing medical discourse would have had little effect.

Women's use of medical discourse in their birth plans seems at once important and a possible impediment to their creating ethical appeals—establishing themselves in their writing as knowledgeable and credible. But medical discourse that is connected to an invocation of their own bodily knowledges and/or experiences of childbirth may function differently. Medical terminology, while not fully persuasive by itself, may hold more rhetorical force when combined with the stories behind and the arguments for various requests. Through such combinations of educational and bodily knowledges, women try to connect with their caregivers on both professional and personal levels, thereby enhancing their ethical appeals.

Ethical Appeals

Each birth plan makes some sort of ethical appeal, but I argue that the most readily effective types are those that invoke previous birth experience to explain or deepen the personal stakes of a given request. Beth and Karen, writing birth plans for their second and third births, respectively, narrate their previous experiences with birth to establish and reinforce this type of ethical appeal. A woman's experience with previous births is important to how her requests are perceived by medical staff. Physicians use the phrase "trial of labor" to describe (attempts at) vaginal birth. A woman who has successfully completed a vaginal birth—having emerged victorious from a previous "trial"—occupies a firmer rhetorical position from which to make requests and demands than a primipara (Latin medical term for "first birth").

In order to convey her specific requests, Beth combines the bullet-point style common in templates with brief but poignant narrative explanations.

She makes pointed requests and backs them up by sharing information from her previous birth. While Beth "would like to avoid tearing," she "would rather have an episiotomy," explaining that she "tore badly last time" and is "scared of that happening again." Beth shares relevant details from the story of her previous birth to draw attention to the experience in her use of "I." Perhaps in part due to these strategies, Beth's birth plan was "followed very closely" for her second and third births (survey). (Of course, her requesting rather than denying certain interventions may also have helped.)

Karen and Sander, who planned a home birth and wrote the birth plan solely in case of hospital transfer, were in a difficult rhetorical position as birth plan authors, one they overcame in part by writing in narrative form. Because home birth is a choice that physicians are often openly hostile to, Karen and Sander carefully establish themselves, from the very first sentence of their birth plan, as Dutch. They explain, "We come from a country where home births are normal and hospital births have a minimum of interventions." By positioning themselves as functioning outside of usual American obstetric practices, not because they are somehow crazy or simply resistant to authority but because birth functions differently where they come from than in usual American obstetric practice, Karen and Sander create an ethical appeal based on experience—experience different from that of their physicians and caregivers. They go on to cite bodily experience with home birth, writing, "We had our first 2 babies at home in the Netherlands and we are planning to have a homebirth again." Like Beth, Karen and Sander establish an ethos of experience to strengthen their rhetorical position in the birth plan and to weaken anticipated resistance to their plan. Because they can tailor their plans based on past experience with birth, Beth and Karen seem to have a certain rhetorical and physical advantage over first-time mothers in preparing for birth.

First-time mothers are not without their own rhetorical strategies, however. Because they cannot rely on past birthing experiences, first-time mothers are perhaps more likely to bolster their ethos through ingratiating themselves to caregivers, a politeness strategy analyzed above. But first-time mothers can and do also rely on educational knowledge, and some also incorporate ethical appeals based on their bodily knowledge, as we see with RH, who writes, "I tend to tense up when I am around people with whom I am not intimately familiar. So, it would be favorable if my husband and I were alone as often as possible." RH's request relies on establishing herself as a woman who knows her body's reaction to particular situations;

she straightforwardly explains the reasons for her request but makes the request itself in the distanced politeness strategy discussed above.

The combination of strategies in RH's request is found in many of the requests—the rhetorical strategies women use overlap and intersect. I have offered one reading of these five birth plans, finding pronouns, politeness strategies, legalese, medical discourse, and ethical appeals to be significant rhetorical features. Alternate readings are possible and suggest the depth and richness of the birth plan as a genre for further exploration. Looking beyond an analysis of the particular rhetorical strategies these women implement, we can begin to see what these birth plans, and the birth plan genre itself, suggest about women's expectations and experiences of rhetorical agency—or the lack thereof—in childbirth and what rhetorical scholars can learn from their rhetorical successes and failures.

CONFRONTING RHETORICAL DISABILITY

Beth is an example of a woman seeking to confront rhetorical disability; she claims agency over her birth and explicitly claims a voice for herself through her birth plan. She writes of her birth plan, "i wanted it to speak for me when I could not speak for myself" (survey). In her online birth story, Beth describes her first birth, telling about being immobilized by the drug (Nubain) she was given. Although she did not object at that time to the drug itself, she was unaware of how drastically it would affect her senses and her ability to communicate. Without her consent and against her wishes, she endured catheterization, vacuum extraction, and her baby's immediate removal from her sight for "routine" procedures. Beth serves as an example of how a woman can be rhetorically disabled through the pain management strategies (one form of technology) administered to her. Beth's birth plan, written for subsequent births as a reaction to this birth, expresses explicit desire to control the application of technology to her birth. Beth uses her writing to reassert bodily authority and to overcome rhetorical disability.

Bodily authority can also, of course, be asserted bodily rather than in writing. Pierre Bourdieu argues in *The Logic of Practice* that "the body believes in what it plays at: it weeps if it mimes grief" (73). In other words, a body will react to its own actions. Bearing a child in an American hospital is a practice saturated with embodied norms, from a woman's location (in the hospital) to her position in that hospital (inferior to staff) to the position of her body (lying on her back in a bed). Such practices have been normalized by doctors and nurses and through countless media images. We can see how a body placed in a position of passivity, in a rhetorical space where it may be voiceless, and in a physical pose shown to be far from conducive for most births (see Arms; Gaskin, *Ina May's Guide*; Goer; Wertz and Wertz) might believe itself to be weak, inferior, and unproductive—and act accordingly. Add to this the numerous technologies brought to bear on the birthing body, and it is not difficult to see why some women feel they must write a birth plan in an effort to insert their agency into this process.

American society (but not all societies—see Jordan, *Birth of Four Cultures*) places much emphasis on the pain of childbirth and alleviating or avoiding that pain; we see childbirth as an event inseparable from pain. Birthing women are not expected to be able to speak—perhaps because language cannot describe the bodily experience of pain (see Scarry 6, 12)—they are not expected to have agency; they are not expected to be rhetorically enabled. By writing birth plans, women seek to triumph over this loss of rhetorical power, but by anticipating this, by writing birth plans and expecting the documents to speak for them, it may be that women are, to a certain extent, participating in their ideological positioning as rhetorically disabled. Recall that RH writes, "If I ask for medical pain relief, please offer encouragement (ex: 'but you're doing so well!') or remind me of non-medical choices such as changing positions." By including in her birth plan a specific request that her oral requests during childbirth essentially be deflected, RH may write herself into a position of rhetorical disability even as she writes to avoid it.

The issue of rhetorical disability is problematic both for women as patients and for doctors as providers. Should doctors and nurses not respond positively (and immediately) to a woman's request for pain medication, they may be excoriated; nonetheless, websites offering birth plan advice note that some women write into their birth plans comments like "no drugs even if I scream for them" (Cuddy), a more extreme and potentially rhetorically disabling request than RH's. Birth attendants faced with a woman screaming for drugs and a piece of paper adamantly refusing drugs must be hard-pressed to determine which path to follow. Suzanne Arms offers one reading of this dilemma, suggesting that a woman screaming for assistance (which may be verbalized as a request for drugs) may need emotional help as much as or more than pharmacological help.

Women who want pain relief—in accepted pharmaceutical forms—can usually get it without words. Anthropologist Brigitte Jordan finds that American women must *enact* pain in order to get pharmaceutical pain relief:

> Since no objective assessment of pain is possible, it is up to the woman to produce the appropriate *display* of the pain experience. . . . The required display of that need not only adds to the comparatively high level of noise and hysteria in American obstetrical wards but must also provide powerful feedback to increase the subjective experience of pain. (*Birth in Four Cultures* 53; my emphasis)

Women whose verbal requests will not be heeded can instead use their bodies to make a rhetorical demonstration of pain, thereby overcoming their rhetorical disability to a certain extent.

That the body speaks, even trumps the voice, at the very moment when the body is supposed to impede the voice may seem to contradict the notion of rhetorical disability; however, it may be that this body language is effective only in acquiring pain medication or other sanctioned assistance. Rhetorical agency is granted the body whose request conforms to Western medical expectations. Women wanting anything outside the norms, however, can get it only *through* words. Women expecting not to be able to use language during birth and anticipating desires they cannot express through gesture write birth plans, as Beth did, to speak for them when they (think they) will not be able to speak for themselves.

Because the experience of childbirth is unique to each birth and widely (even wildly) variant in terms of perceived pain and success of pain management strategies, women may not be able to definitively decide their preferences prior to the experience. While the plan may offer a preview of women's desires and expectations and may reinforce her expression of those desires when she "cannot speak," it cannot adjust as her needs and desires might or replace on-the-spot decision making.[9] Despite these challenges, the illusion of control a birth plan offers is appealing to many women and is the primary reason women like Beth write birth plans—but, as I argue below, it may not be the primary benefit of writing birth plans.

While of debatable value as a tool enabling women to resist particular interventions, control their births, or overcome rhetorical disability, I argue that the birth plan has tremendous value as an educational tool. Through writing birth plans, women embody the philosophy of writing to learn. Writing a birth plan requires research, which leads to knowledge, which can lead to more complete, less didactic interactions with birth attendants before birth, when issues of time and rhetorical disability are less likely to interfere with communication. Birth plans are complex rhetorical documents. The choices birth plan writers make go far beyond the boxes they might check on a template; their grammatical, rhetorical, and content choices have material and lasting effects—even when the plan is not followed. Women writing birth plans write themselves into particular understandings of birth. In doing so, they simultaneously write themselves into particular understandings of their relation to knowledge, to medicine, and to society.

The birth plan is a paradoxical document. It seeks to guarantee a particular form of care largely by disrupting what the expected birth attendants are likely to see as the best form of care. The birth plan calls attention to itself as a document that raises precise expectations, even as it may overtly recognize the futility of having precise expectations for a rather unpredictable event.

In order to write birth plans, women must learn, construct, and usually challenge ideological meanings of childbirth in our society. Julia's experience replacing her caregiver at the eleventh hour (or ninth month) represents a successful implementation of the birth plan as an educational tool. In birth plans, women display various forms of knowledge gained, from the embodied or experiential to the educated, scientific, or medical. Although I have presented the birth plan as chock-full of interesting rhetorical tactics, I have also shown that these strategies often do not produce the material results women seek. That said, however, I do see significant potential for this document. The birth plan may never result in an idealized birth, in part because birth can never be precisely planned, regardless of the location or attendants. While physicians may share with midwives and patients the idea of a perfect birth—one where, as former obstetrician Judith Brysk puts it, they can "sit on their hands" until the baby's head crowns, at which point they would "throw on some gloves" and catch the baby—doctors are unlikely to experience the epistemological shift that would be required for them to avoid intervening when their training would lead them to do so. Also, although many women resist medicalized birthing techniques, more than 99 percent of American women choose to give birth in hospitals (Martin et al., "Births: Final Data for 2004"; Mitford), where such techniques are expected and routinized.

In their efforts to write birth plans, women educate themselves about pregnancy and birth, learning about themselves as consumers, patients, and possessors of unpredictable bodies. Just as women can consult myriad birth plan templates online, they can also find advice, support groups, and information about issues such as miscarriage and stillbirth.

The birth plan holds the most promise for women—and for their care providers—as an educational tool rather than as a prescriptive contract. It helps women educate themselves about birth, but it also helps them educate their care providers about their preferences, which can lead to important changes. When women resist certain procedures, responses from physicians and attendants vary. Women's online birth narratives suggest that some doctors and staff attempt to accommodate requests, but not consistently. They also note that support for their requests can change as new birth attendants take over their care after shift changes. Other attendants become annoyed, some going so far as to express the hope or expectation that a woman with a birth plan will end up with a C-section ("Birth Plans"). Other care providers, however, when confronted over time with women's birth plans, may wonder why women write them and what interventions they are resisting and may come to question why those interventions are performed in the first place. Such change has happened before: women consistently resisted the practices of pubic shaving and routine enemas, which began in hospitals in the 1890s (Wertz and Wertz). Such procedures had become routine by the 1950s before practices changed in the late 1970s and early 1980s (Brysk; Mitford). Because of women's consistent vocal resistance, researchers performed studies that found these two practices "didn't make a [positive] difference," says Brysk: not only did they not prevent infection and defecation during delivery, as intended, they actually increased the chances of both. And many women hated them. These procedures are no longer routine.

Vocal resistance led to change, resulting in a minirevolution in birth practices. Michel Foucault says, "It is doubtless the strategic codification of . . . resistance that makes a revolution possible" (*History* 96). Birth plans, a written form of resistance, work together with women's voices to codify particular resistances. As in the shaving and enema examples above, women's resistance, when deployed consistently over time, can create change. The birth plan may hold little effect as an individual document seeking control over one woman's birth experience, but it can have value as an educational tool for individual women. Additionally, the collective power of birth plans, shared over time with medical staff, might lead to enhanced understandings of birth and real changes in birth practices. The fact that change has happened in the past, not for individual women at the time of their vocalized resistance but for women later, supports the argument that women's assertions of feminist rhetorical agency, even if not successful for themselves or in a particular moment, can nevertheless evoke change.

Birth plans are a prime example of writing in the world serving multiple functions: they instigate birth and pregnancy education; they serve as a repository of birth information for women and medical staff; they display numerous rhetorical strategies; they facilitate discussion and decision making; and they allow women to assert their rhetorical agency to (attempt to) intervene in the usual hierarchy of patient-doctor relationships, representing a significant and political resistance to that assumed authority. While the birth plan can certainly serve as an example of rhetorical failure, this analysis demonstrates that rhetorical failure can also be read as, and thereby transformed into, rhetorical possibility.

CHAPTER FOUR

HOSTiNG BiRTH

Birth and Birth Stories over Time and Online

Ame's birth story, posted on *Plomp.com*, a website devoted solely to sharing birth stories, refers to a birth that didn't go according to plan (an outcome readers of chapters 2 and 3 will not find particularly surprising):

> My original plan included no pain meds, no IV if possible, no shave, no episiotomy, none of the "usual" stuff . . . Around 3:30 am Anne did another exam and . . . we decided to break my water. Well, that's when things got off track . . . I ended up getting an IV put in . . . I had an episiotomy, a few 1st degree tears, a 2nd degree and a 3rd degree . . . I am most proud that I stuck to my no pain meds.

Ame doesn't simply explain what went wrong, however; she also asserts joy and redemption about what went right—"I am most proud that I stuck to my no pain meds." Ame tells a story of some triumph in the face of adversity. She describes where she had agency and reclaims rhetorical agency over her birth through her story.

The website where Ame shared her story, like others devoted to such sharing, illustrates the role the Internet can play in distributing feminist rhetorical agency. These sites enable a vast group of women to disclose intimate details about their births to an even vaster group of readers preparing for or interested in birth. While authors and scholars as diverse as Cherrie Moraga, Isabel Allende, Suzanne Arms, and Robbie Davis-Floyd have written about their personal experiences with childbirth and motherhood, it is only recently that contemporary women who are not "writers" have been able to write and share their experiences with the public. These ordinary women's online birth stories bring the experiences of everyday women into anyone's ken, and they not only entertain but educate. They also reveal aspects of women's experiences and attitudes toward childbirth, motherhood, and their roles in society.

Unlike Ame, Gabriela experienced no adversity, but like Ame, she also conveys triumph as she harnesses an online space to make sweeping pronouncements and overtly political statements in her story at *UnassistedChildbirth.com*:

> I don't depend on doctors, Nestle bottles, or the goodness of the establishment. Many women are blinded by "false liberation" and the crazy run for money, thinking that motherhood is slavery. Wrong. The woman who has homebirth and breastfeeds a long time, is using the power that Nature gave her. She is free and powerful.

Gabriela writes confidently, secure in her beliefs, in her choices, and in what sets her apart—and, to her, above—women and mothers who make different choices. Joseph's mother, writing on *Childbirth.org*, also speaks frankly of her personal experience:

> Joseph was born on Oct 6, 1995 and at that time I didn't know there was such a web-site devoted to this type of issue; it would have been a great help. . . . The hospital and doctors dealt with my physical problems quite effectively but there was no emotional support in my hospital and no information about what I had gone through.

Joseph's mother makes explicit her gratitude for the space and freedom to write. She brings the emotional needs of birthing mothers to the fore and illustrates the personal benefit of online birth stories and the information they and their host sites make available. These three women, writing on three different childbirth and parenting websites, provide a glimpse into the variety and significance of online birth stories and the way those reflect and can be affected by their location.

This chapter provides a "thick description" of key textual, visual, and commercial features of the five childbirth and parenting websites in this study[1] and of their influences on the stories they solicit and host (Geertz). Each site's owners solicit and host these stories for a variety of purposes, which include (but are not limited to) the distribution of everyday women's experiential birth knowledge. I argue that this distribution provides unprecedented opportunities but also that the distribution is not always straightforward or unimpeded; by influencing or placing conditions on women's birth stories, these sites can limit, as well as spread, feminist rhetorical agency.

As previous chapters have shown, childbirth is extensively shaped by cultural norms and often dramatically affected by technological mediation. The websites examined here reflect and often reinscribe cultural norms surrounding childbirth, but not all sites agree about what those norms are or should be. By examining the ways the websites provide women a promise or glimpse of connection, invite and use women's birth stories, inculcate notions of consumerism, and demonstrate beliefs about pregnancy and women's bodies, I show that the websites' words and images establish, affirm, and (less often) challenge childbirth's dominant norms, discourses, and cultural scripts in the contemporary United States.

BIRTH STORIES' PURPOSES AND CONVENTIONS

Birth stories are often untold and unwritten. Oral narratives do exist but tend to circulate among small groups of women, such as at baby showers and in maternity wards and childbirth classes. Written narratives, too, have tended to have particular, small audiences, such as those of letters and diaries (Huff; Leavitt, *Brought to Bed*). Such stories have particular conventions: rhetorician Cynthia Huff, for example, describes a Victorian diarist's birth story entry by noting its similarity to other birth story entries: "Like other diarists, Lady Brougham notes when her pains began, how they progressed and when the birth occurred, as well as who attended it and where it took place" (129).

These conventions (time, progress, location, attendants) are also present in the excerpts of diaries and letters that historian Judith Leavitt uses in *Brought to Bed*, her study of early American women's childbirth experiences, suggesting the birth story is a genre with fairly established content expectations. Women who today share birth stories via email and blogs and on childbirth and parenting websites depend upon traditional incarnations of the birth story even as they alter that genre in this new medium of the Internet. They share details that echo those of earlier diarists and letter writers, providing careful chronologies and lists of characters involved.

Occasionally birth story authors defy those expectations or conventions of the genre. Laurie, who explicitly writes a counternarrative, explains: "You may note that there are a few things missing from this birth story. No one told me when I was in labor. No one checked or recorded my dilation, effacement, or station. No one told me when or where to sit up, lie down, eat, drink, or pee." ("Angelica's Birth Story"). Laurie's careful reckoning of absent but expected details speaks to her understanding of the genre as well as to her understanding of hospital versus home births. Laurie writes out of an expectation that people reading will be familiar with (hospital) birth and birth stories, invoking and lightly challenging her unknown audience.

Some birth story authors echo a typically oral form of birth story: the "horror stories" that strangers often inflict on pregnant women, which seem to serve a disciplinary function in that they attempt to ensure women's fears of childbirth. At my own baby shower, one relative told her "horror story" of a long, painful labor with many complications, but another relative quickly countered with the tale of her own short, almost painless natural birth experience. The two women nearly shouted, each offering sweeping pronouncements on the nature of childbearing, dismissing the other's experience and advice. Their stories fit handily into the two dominant views of childbirth, one finding labor an uplifting and sometimes even painless "natural" experience, the other finding that "same" experience excruciating, painful, and unbearable, grateful for medical attention and intervention.

While horror stories are prevalent, what Tess Cosslett calls the "primitive woman" story is less commonly told by modern American women, although websites such as *UnassistedChildbirth.com* explicitly provide a space for just such stories. While the horror story tends to be couched as advice based on lived experience, so, too, are the natural childbirth stories; while one story relies on fear, discourages deviation from a "norm," and encourages cooperation with birth attendants, the other relies on what might be called faith, encourages deviation from what has become a norm (medicalized birth), and advises trust in bodily knowledge. The two story types are at opposite ends of the wide range of stories women remember and share online and offline.

MEDIATION AND REMEDIATION

Writing birth stories online allows women to mediate their birth experiences, giving them a way to link memory with expression. Whether women become "victims" or "victors" after giving birth is determined by three factors, including "the mother's social context, the medicalization of the birth, and the *mediation of maternal feelings* about this" (Oakley 176; my emphasis). In the next chapter, I show how some women come to avoid "victim" status by writing and posting birth stories, but beyond mediation on the emotional level, the stories qualify as remediations: reformulations of birth itself and of birth stories told in other forms, through other media.

In their landmark essay "Remediation" (and subsequent book of the same title), Jay David Bolter and Richard Grusin argue that "all current media function as remediators and that remediation offers us a means of interpreting the work of earlier media as well" (345). An awareness of the generic components of traditional birth stories informs my argument that their online descendants constitute remediations. Bolter and Grusin explicate three instances of the "double logic" of remediation: remediation is the mediation of mediation; remediation is the inseparability of mediation and reality; and remediation is reform (346). In each of these senses, online birth stories qualify as remediated.

I see women's appropriation of this new medium to share these stories as enacting a move toward reform of childbirth itself more than as an effort "to refashion or rehabilitate other media" (346). Birth stories as remediation constitute a type of reform that includes but is far more extensive than that of the media itself. Bolter and Grusin allow that "remediation can also imply reform in a social or political sense" (351), and it is in this sense that I apply the term here. The digitized birth story, because of its accessibility, accomplishes far more than traditional forms of birth stories.

Women's consumption and production of online birth stories may be an attempt to recover, virtually, components of what was once a shared, rather than a mostly solitary, experience. American women's experience of birth today is vastly different from their experience of birth even two hundred years ago; as their birth experience changes, so do their needs as writers and as readers. Childbirth changes go far beyond the obvious technological advances and the shift in dominant location to hospitals. Women today rarely attend one another's births and also have far fewer children than in generations past.[2] As Carol Downer explains, "The normal human experience of childbirth . . . has been entirely removed from daily life, so that most of us have no direct knowledge of it" (qtd. in Treichler 121). Important is the detail that childbirth once was woven into the fabric of women's everyday lives.

FROM SOCIAL BIRTH COTERIE TO VIRTUAL BIRTH COTERIE?

In colonial times in North America, in addition to a midwife, a birthing woman's friends and relatives would come to the home to "provide comfort and practical aid" (Wertz and Wertz 2).[3] Richard W. Wertz and Dorothy C. Wertz explain:

> The normal practice was to make birth itself a social event for a coterie of women, whom the husband often assembled. . . . Birth presented an important, perhaps the primary, occasion for female solidarity. Women

> could help in practical ways at birth, but they attended also . . . *to share their own knowledge and experiences of birth, and to prepare themselves for their own future deliveries.* (4–5; my emphasis)

While women once observed and participated in birth "as a social event" before and during their own childbearing years, gaining significant observational and participatory experience with the process and with different women's ways of handling different births, women today are rather inexperienced with birth. They have little or no individual bodily experience and even less collective observational experience to draw on.[4]

To redress their lack of birth knowledge absorbed through experience, modern American women seek some sort of virtual educational experience in preparation. Many women turn not only to published texts for information, of which there are many today,[5] but also to the Internet. Online, everyday women both learn from and educate other women. Survey respondent PrettyMomma writes that she read online birth stories "as a way of gaining some 'experience' in addition to the informal education I had received from written works by midwives and obstetricians" (survey).

Birth narratives presented online, where any women with access can read them, along with the online support groups often housed at the same sites, operate for some women as a substitute for the experience of physical communities. Lorrie sums up this sentiment in describing why she shared her birth story online: "I remember being very alone when I first had my son and then daughter as my friends were all at work during the day and my online support while I was pregnant and nursing was very important to me" (survey). When Lorrie decided to post her story, she was "thinking of others like [her], who didn't have support from women friends who knew what to expect." Women like Lorrie remediate the genre of the birth story, changing it from a private tale to a public source of information and support.

Women seeking information and support online seem to find it through reading birth stories: women I surveyed describe having benefited from reading stories on these sites in preparation for birth; many hope that contributing their own stories will in turn help other women. All survey respondents had read stories on the sites before they posted their own. Lauren subscribes to the reciprocal expectation; she wrote her online birth story "because I had read so many other stories that I found so helpful that I thought I should contribute my own" (survey). Slimgirl156 writes, "I added my story because there is so much unknown while you are preg I found it helpful knowing there were others out there who felt the same twinges, pains, etc. as me. I wanted new moms-to-be to know that there is help out there and not to be afraid to ask or seek it out" (survey). Slimgirl156 not only shared her birth story online but also participated in online chat groups devoted to birth. While not all birth story authors join chat groups or electronic mailing lists, many women express a desire to form some sort of e-relationship with other women based on their pregnancy and birth experiences.

Reading and writing stories appear to benefit women, but the imagined ideal seems to be to create the opportunity for interactive community (even though that community is rarely actually in evidence in the Web 1.0 atmosphere of the five websites I examined for this study), an impulse that helps to establish the online birth story as remediated. Beyond contributing to communities by submitting stories, some women hope to form communities by forging email connections with authors and readers. Websites that provide story authors' email addresses open up the possibility that readers might contact these experienced women to ask questions and further discuss their stories. Some mothers write this invitation directly into their stories, a convention of the genre examined in the next chapter, while others simply permit the site to provide their address as a link. (It is important to note that these pre–Web 2.0 sites provided no opportunity for comments or interaction; they anticipate that possibility, however.) The presence of email addresses suggests a further distinction between online birth stories and those encountered in letters and diaries. Because women have the option—at least the perceived option—of near-immediate interaction with the writer, they can participate in an exchange perhaps beneficial to both reader and writer. This difference highlights a potentially transformative aspect of the online remediation of the birth story genre, because the medium of the Internet permits such interactional results.

While celebrating the possibility of connection and interaction, however, the reality is that while the story authors, readers, and websites seem to expect these ideals to come to fruition, these idealistic expectations are not well-supported by the sites and are thwarted in various ways. Over time, women's email addresses change and websites provide no forwarding addresses; websites move and delete stories or go through redesigns that disappear or replace some stories; and, as we see in the case of *Plomp.com*, websites can go offline altogether. Here the limitations of the communicative promise of the web-based birth story are revealed, that promise forever unfulfilled. With *Plomp.com* in particular, the remediation leads to a loss of text; as with a library fire, most readers can no longer access the stories. True, savvy web-users might visit the *Internet Archive Wayback Machine* to find a favorite birth story from *Plomp.com*, but this seems unlikely, and certainly no new readers will find the site. The remediation of the birth story, then, is only as successful as each host site; if the site dies, so, essentially, do the stories.[6]

Sites offer some promise of connection by including women's email addresses (Table 4.1), but women's abilities to use that information to successfully form virtual coterie is limited in multiple ways: by the lack of stable connectivity; by the fact that women in American society typically have only a few children, so most are present at these sites only for a limited time with no chance to reconnect; and because the stories are inert, unchanging, within a stable textual frame. In a Web 2.0 context, women would be able to post comments back and forth on stories, breaking the textual frame and, to use Susan Wells's appropriation of the term "metalepsis," "enlist[ing] the reader in the construction of knowledge" (100), thereby strengthening readers' belief in the knowledge of the text. Such construction and exchange would produce a new layer of knowledge and connection, but this connection was not available to story writers and story readers in my study; the stories' effect on readers is not visible to other readers. Even without actual connectivity, however, the promise of connection still seems to serve a valuable purpose for women writing and reading these stories.

COMMODIFYING WOMEN'S EXPERIENCES

As Table 4.1 shows, I categorize the sites into two types: corporate and noncorporate. I make these distinctions based on sites' uses of advertising and on the ways they copyright women's birth stories. The "corporate" sites (*BirthStories.com*, *Childbirth.org*, and *TheLaborofLove.com*) link to numerous commercial sites and advertise everything from software to sunglasses. *BirthStories.com* and *TheLaborofLove.com* are also owned by corporations, *BirthStories.com* by Disney and *TheLaborofLove.com* by Earth's Magic, Inc. *Childbirth.org*, by contrast, was created and originally owned by one woman, Robin Elise Weiss, but fits with the other corporate sites because of its extensive advertisements and ways of appropriating birth stories. The noncorporate sites, Karen Plomp's *Plomp.com* and Laura Shanley's *UnassistedChildbirth.com* (also called "Bornfree!"), have no apparent corporate tie-ins and minimal external advertising, though both link to their own

Table 4.1. *Email Connection and Site Status of Five Childbirth and Parenting Websites*

	Email address availability	Email address information	Site status	Type of site	Registered site owner*
BirthStories.com	With some stories	Link from mother's name, but some links go to a generic BirthStories.com website.	Live	Corporate	iParenting, LLC (in 2005); Network Solutions, LLC, a subsidiary of Disney Enterprises (by 2010)
Childbirth.org	No	n/a	Partially revived	Corporate	Robin Elise Weiss
TheLaborofLove.com	With some stories	Link from mother's name	Live	Corporate	Earth's Magic, Inc.
Plomp.com	With a majority of stories	Link from mother's name or "author"; some addresses do not appear as links. For example, name@school.edu would appear like this: name at school dot edu.	Defunct/ offline	Non-corporate	Karen Plomp
UnassistedChildbirth.com	With very few stories	Link from author's name	Live	Non-corporate	Laura Shanley

* *According to "WHOIS Behind That Domain?"*

online stores or request donations. (The current iteration of Shanley's site includes external Google ads, but at the time of the survey the site was free of external advertisements; Plomp's site, now offline, never had external ads.)

Beyond advertising, what is significant about the distinction between corporate and noncorporate sites is the ways they take legal ownership of the stories submitted to them. All three sites I call corporate expressly copyright women's stories. Beyond merely "hosting" the stories, the corporate sites use women's birth stories as a profit-making opportunity. Websites optimize search engine results by creating content that will attract visitors and encourage people to link to their sites. Birth stories on childbirth and parenting websites serve identical purposes in terms of readership. The corporate sites have a financial interest in collecting and offering birth stories, but each of the corporate sites makes a legal claim not only to collect and offer but to *own* the stories.

TheLaborofLove.com makes use of boilerplate legal language:

> Disclosure and Use of Your Communications—Postings to this site and electronic mail delivered to The Labor of Love are not confidential and The Labor of Love shall not be liable for any use or disclosure thereof. All communications and other materials . . . you send to this site or to The Labor of Love by electronic mail are, and shall remain, the sole and exclusive property of The Labor of Love and may be used by The Labor of Love for any purpose whatsoever, commercial or otherwise, without compensation. ("Terms of Use")

Not only does the site claim the right to use "all communications and other materials," but it also claims all such information as its own "sole and exclusive property." *Childbirth.org* also copyrights all stories and offers the statement "All rights reserved." At *Childbirth.org*, however, the site makes no use of legal language. No section of the site explains any policies on terms of use. *BirthStories.com* offers this explanation: "If you submit content to our site . . . we own all rights to that information and can use it in any form, online, print or other" ("Privacy Policy Statement"). By 2010 the site had updated the language to read, "By submitting your story, you agree to allow BirthStories.com and iParenting Media to use your story or excerpts thereof. For more details, please see our Disclaimer [link] and read our Terms of Use [link]" ("Birth Stories"). The focus here is on their rights to *use* the stories as they see fit; the meaning of "all rights" is somewhat unclear, at least to this reader.

These sites protect their commercial interests by establishing that the stories sent to them are legally theirs to use as they please for posting and advertising purposes. Only *TheLaborofLove.com* seems also to nullify women's own rights to the stories, with the phrase "sole and exclusive property." This aspect of birth story remediation and online publication is perhaps less empowering to women than others. The shift in birth story ownership from women to host site speaks to the complex nature of remediation and online publication.

Neither of the two noncorporate sites takes copyright ownership of women's stories. At the time of my survey, *Plomp.com* provided a simple place for women to share and read birth stories. The site's home page, titled "Birth Stories" (with several exclamation points), was born of Karen Plomp's sincere interest in childbirth. Plomp's own home-birth stories—a mother of seven, Plomp had six home births—make an implicit argument against hospital births, but she offers no explicit agenda for birth and no judgments of the women whose narratives she tends. She offers her reasons for soliciting birth stories and maintaining the site simply:

> *Why did I set up this page?* Well, I really like to read birth stories, and I know I am not the only one who enjoys reading them :-) . . . I am part of the June 96 moms [link] list and it all started with setting up a page for them, also with a lot of their birth stories. I enjoyed doing that and decided to do the same for other people. ("Birth Stories!!!")

Plomp's straightforward position is that she posts birth stories to satisfy her own desire to read them and to do others a good turn simultaneously. In addition to this explicit reasoning—kindly sharing stories and enabling others to also—this site and others like it allow women to simulate, in effect, communities of the past where women attended one another's births, knew the intimate physical details and signs of good, bad, and even ugly birthing situations, and felt capable of giving birth. *Plomp.com*, like all birth story websites, allows women to remediate their birth stories, to access and learn from other birth stories, and, in some cases, to question and bond with other women in similar situations. Or at least it did until it went offline.

As media and their content evolve and adapt, so too do understandings of intellectual property; in this case, women's experiences become commodities. Certainly scholars in the humanities have been well trained to view commodification as problematic, at best. And at first glance, websites' commodification of women's experiences could be read as damaging to women, or at least to their ability to use their experiences and stories for their own agency or for their own financial, intellectual, emotional, or other purposes—and it may be. But the commodification through copyright also may have a positive effect, in that the sites that copyright stories remain online, perhaps in part because of the financial stability lent by taking ownership of the stories. The only site of the five in this study that made no mention of copyright whatsoever, *Plomp.com*, is also the only site that is no longer online. While not definitive, the website's demise hints that commodification may actually have benefits for the survival of these stories, and thus for the women who gain feminist rhetorical agency from writing and/or reading them.

The stories on all five sites provide searchable, already collected, often labeled archives of scores of birth stories that any woman can access, and as the next chapter demonstrates, these stories and sites are quite important to women's understandings of and acceptance of a wide range of childbirth experiences. Reading birth stories helps women prepare for and reminisce about childbirth, and writing birth stories for online publication helps women come to new understandings of birth, of their own agency, and of their potential to help other women. These benefits are many, so while the commodification of the stories suggests the corporate sites' less-than-beneficent intentions, one alternative, a site that may not survive, complicates a kneejerk anti-commodification stance. Ownership helps ensure a site's stability, which enhances the connective possibility of the site and allows women continued access to the stories.

CATEGORIES AS INVENTION CONTROL AND CONSUMER TARGETING

All sites categorize the birth stories they host in some way, most by birth "type." The sites' categorizations, on one level, simply assist readers in finding a birth story they would like to read, but on another level, the categorizations serve as terministic screens, to use Kenneth Burke's terminology: they reflect realities of the birth stories, but they also necessarily select only partial aspects of those realities and simultaneously deflect other realities, challenging readers' full appreciation of any woman's birth story. (And of course each woman's word choices in each story act as further terministic screens, which perpetuate these acts of reflection, selection, and deflection for readers.)

The corporate sites tend to organize stories by birth type (Table 4.2). In addition to the writers' own titles for their birth stories, which are sometimes as simple as "Joey's Birth Story," the corporate sites all categorize the stories, often based on medical intervention(s), number child, and location. *BirthStories.com* provides a search box for finding stories with keywords, offers a "featured story," and organizes the rest by its twelve categories, while *TheLaborofLove.com* and *Childbirth.org* both provide readers with two or more options. *TheLaborofLove.com* offers two groupings in addition to its own categorized lists: the five "latest" and the five "most popular" birth stories, encouraging readers to continue to visit the site to find new stories and to read those made popular by others. *Childbirth.org* shows the most explicit audience accommodation of the three corporate sites, explaining, "After listening to our readers, we found that many of you read a collection of stories during your lunch hour," so the site now offers two options: numbered collections—five stories of varying type grouped together—and stories categorized by type. Most of the stories also have author-created titles. Site visitors, then, to the three corporate sites are guided to particular stories through the different ways sites highlight them and via site-specific categorizations.

These categorizations, when required as selections prior to posting, serve as powerful ingredients for what Burke calls "improvisational freedom":

> Insofar as there can be cycles of terms that imply one another, and all such terms can be translated into terms of either images or ideas, and any such idea can serve as a point of departure, providing a perspective peculiar to its particular point of view, the sheer range of such possibilities sets up the conditions for an ingredient of improvisational "freedom" in men's [*sic*] powers of symbolic action. (*Language* 62)

Through the predetermined, often medically focused categorizations of the corporate sites, as well as in the ways they solicit and guide women's birth stories (about which more below), sites can limit women's access to and awareness of the fullest range of birth experiences and possibilities, even as the stories they provide can also help broaden women's knowledge and perspective. The sites can even delimit what women can write about the births they have experienced, which could limit their ability to achieve fulfillment of a pursuit of retroactive agency. As Burke suggests, the range of possibilities for terms leads to improvisational freedom; conversely, when both reading and writing are contracted or constrained by terms chosen by

Table 4.2. *Categorizations and Descriptions of Birth Stories*

	BirthStories.com	*Childbirth.org*	*TheLaborofLove.com*	*Plomp.com*	*UnassistedChildbirth.com*
Ways of organizing/ describing/ accessing stories	By category: interventions or birth "type"	By category: interventions or birth "type" Also groups five most recently submitted stories—not selected by type	By category: interventions or birth "type" Also groups five "latest" and five "most popular" stories	Year (1970–2004), then birthday, name(s), and individualized list of characteristics	Title, name, and descriptive phrase, usually opening with positive adjective
Categories or sample descriptions	• First baby • First baby after a loss • Second or more • Home births • Natural births • Extremely fast • Induced labor • Multiples • Scheduled C-section • Complicated pregnancy • Young mothers • Premature babies	• Cesarean birth stories • Complicated birth stories • Home-birth stories • Medicated birth stories • Unmedicated birth stories • Vaginal birth after Cesarean birth stories	• Home births • Hospital births • Birth center births • Natural births • Multiple births • C-section births • VBAC births • Complicated births • Premature births • Young mothers • First baby • Siblings present	• "2004, [birthday,] then: Lupus, Cytotec, Pitocin induction epidural, baby in NICU. 2nd kid" • "Birthcenter. Waterbirth. Unmedicated. 1st kid."	• Beautiful waterbirth by the fireplace • Empowering birth during a thunderstorm • A speeding birth on the Autobahn • Sensual birth in Argentina

others and when women select terms among given options rather than create their own, that "improvisational 'freedom'" is somewhat thwarted (62).

The noncorporate sites differ in their categorization techniques. Each of the sites operates with its own particular agenda, revealed in part by those categorizations. For the corporate sites, that agenda is to drive advertisements; given that scenario, limits on improvisational freedom (part of what makes the online birth story remediated from other genres of birth stories) can be seen as ways of targeting consumers. On the noncorporate sites, by contrast, reaching "consumers" is not the goal. For Shanley, the explicit agenda of her site is to increase awareness and acceptance of unassisted childbirth—thus her site limits the location and style of childbirth stories. Aside from that (admittedly large) delimitation, Shanley places no improvisational limits on the birth stories her site houses. The vast lists of medical interventions woven into the corporate sites' categories, for example, are absent at *UnassistedChildbirth.com*, which provides only one type of story (all births described there are unassisted, therefore unmedicated, and usually at home)—or perhaps two, if intentionally versus unintentionally unassisted births are considered separately. Her categories are not so much categories, then, as they are descriptive, evocative titles.

Plomp.com goes yet another route, including more information for each category than any other site. It is the only one of the five sites to categorize by year and to always also include the child's birthday. The site provides readers with hundreds of diverse birthing stories dating back to 1970 (the single story from that year is the first listed—of a boy named, perhaps appropriately for a first, Adam). Karen Plomp lists brief attributes of each story within the year grouping; only after choosing a year can readers see the short list of descriptive details such as medical interventions, outcomes, and number child. *Plomp.com*, then, seems the most "improvisationally free" and the most open to various routes of reclaiming agency, given Plomp's stated interest in simply reading and providing space for others to read and share birth stories.

MORE INVENTIONAL CONTROL AND CONSUMER TARGETING

I turn now to an examination of the different ways each of these websites invites readers to share their stories. These invitations are more complicated than one might imagine and affect not only the existence of a story on a site but also its content, structure, and appearance—which in turn affect the types of audiences drawn to the stories. While every site in this study offers readers the chance to share their birth stories, the language and form of the invitations range from offering general content guidance to delimiting what women can, or "should," include. The invitations, then, set parameters and attempt to control women's invention of their birth stories.

Women's inventional processes as they write their birth stories are, or can be, affected by the ways each site invites submissions. Below I examine those invitations, seeking a better understanding of each of the sites and their influence on women's childbirth narratives, beginning with *Plomp.com*. Given Karen Plomp's straightforward explanation of her rationale for hosting the stories, readers might expect her site to offer women the most inventional freedom and the least inventional constraints, and indeed it does. With no editorializing or further directions, she simply includes this sentence: "If you want to contribute your birth story, please send it to me at plomp@together.net." ("Birth Stories!!!"). Plomp offers the most unfettered invitations to women seeking to assert feminist rhetorical agency over their births and stories. (Plomp also always invites readers to share pictures, also via email, as does *UnassistedChildbirth.com*, but none of the corporate sites provide that option.)

Because each site's popularity relies at least in part on its birth story traffic and on women seeking to submit stories after having benefited from reading them, it is somewhat surprising that the sites do not consistently *accept* stories, even while providing pages and links suggesting they do, and that the invitations to submit stories are sometimes deeply embedded in the sites. *BirthStories.com* is the only corporate site that has consistently accepted stories; from May 2000 through November 2005, the site included an enthusiastic invitation on its index page, complete with exclamation points, a handwriting-like font, and graphics of pen and paper.[7] The image of a pad and pen was somewhat ironic, but the image suggests that the site's authors recognized the genre remediation they were requesting by asking women to type into a computer, for public consumption, what would traditionally be part of a handwritten letter or private journal entry. The image operates as a skeuomorph, "a design feature that is no longer functional in itself but that refers back to a feature that was functional at an earlier time. . . . Skeuomorphs testify to the social or psychological necessity for innovation to be tempered by replication" (Hayles 17). The skeuomorph hails writers, beckoning them with the familiar and the simple.

Beyond the graphic connection to past incarnations of the birth story, the invitation on *BirthStories.com* to write also describes desired story details, or "things to think about when sharing your story," which include such aspects of birth as "the duration of the various stages of your labor, how you felt during the experiences, how you reacted to and coped with labor and the birth, as well as the baby's gender, weight, and condition" ("Post Your Story").

The 2011 version of the site provides more sophisticated graphics[8] than the pen and paper image but maintains the same invitation, although the list of "things to think about" is prefaced with "We'd love for you to share your story with us—and when your story appears, share the link with your friends and family" ("Birth Stories"). The site encourages women to share their birth stories with people they already know by sending them to this corporate site to read them—generating traffic for the site. This site asks for the author's first name and requests an email address, which will be kept private. At least in this iteration, the site neither provides women a space to share their stories with their full names nor allows readers to contact the authors. The site explicitly deflects a connective possibility for the stories' writers and readers and denies writers the agency that their full names and the chance to connect with readers might enable.

One particularly interesting and politically provocative aspect of *Birth-Stories.com*'s invitations to write is the word "gender" (where readers might expect "sex") in multiple iterations of the site. The use of this term here may attempt to support a view like Judith Butler's that "gender ought not to be conceived merely as the cultural inscription of meaning on a pregiven sex (a juridical conception); gender must also designate the very apparatus of production whereby the sexes themselves are established" (7). The word "gender" here may suggest a certain feminist bent to the website, making a subtle political statement. (It may also, however, suggest that the authors are uncomfortable with the word "sex," which would imply a quite different political stance.) As these websites, and the birth stories appearing on them, participate in the construction of gender, they also participate in the construction of other received "truths": truths about childbirth, women, knowledge, and medicine.

Besides asking for the "gender," the writing advice and details requested here are fairly traditional, both in terms of birth and generic expectations for written birth stories. Such stories consistently note how much time labor takes (or is given), the woman's experience of labor and birth, and basic information on the baby's sex and condition at birth. These directions offer authors a certain amount of rhetorical agency and inventional freedom even as they recommend topics; for example, they make no suggestion that women write about attendants' decisions. That attendants' decisions, and women's (often negative) reactions to them, are regular and significant aspects of birth stories on all five sites suggests one change from the earlier birth stories, which seem to have been more likely to describe the events without second-guessing attendants' decisions (Huff; Leavitt, *Brought to Bed*). This might reflect women's reduced control over their labors and deliveries (Wertz and Wertz; Leavitt, *Brought to Bed*; Borst); however, it might also be an issue of consumerism.

While none of the sites suggest in their invitations to write that women share or post their birth stories as an outlet for describing an unsavory consumer experience, this purpose nonetheless asserts itself frequently, particularly in the stories shared at the corporate sites included in this study. Modern American women are treated as procreative customers throughout their pregnancies by medical staff, insurance companies, websites, and the public. They are told they have choices and are encouraged to exercise their rights, but these rights may extend only so far as choosing attendants or locations and not to exercising the control they expect to have over birth itself, as we saw with women's experiences with birth plans in chapters 2 and 3. Disappointment over birth experiences leads some women to react as any dissatisfied customer might: writing angry letters and stories, filing lawsuits, and steering others away from the source of their dissatisfaction. Stories at all three corporate sites reveal similar issues women have with control, acceptance, and resistance to the medicalization of their births; what we find, then, is that women complain about a (bad) consumer experience of birth at sites that themselves treat them as consumers.

The corporate sites consistently anticipate readers-as-consumers, regularly placing advertisements on the pages that "solicit" stories, even while those solicitations are not live. For example, while from at least November 2003 through July 2010, neither *TheLaborofLove.com* nor *Childbirth.org* accepted new stories, readers at *Childbirth.org* nevertheless encountered a link asking, "Would [you] like to know how to have your story included?," a link that for years remained live, complete with missing subject, but led to a page stating, "We are not currently accepting birth stories." This page (in various iterations over time), however failed in its overt purpose, has remained a lively commercial location: readers of the 2007 version, by following the links prominent at the top of the page, could purchase birth announcements or a film about doulas; a glance at the left side of the page revealed the diversity of topics a woman might explore and other items she might buy as she perused this site.

The specific offerings have changed as the site has been updated; by 2011, although the site itself was still not accepting birth stories, a linked invitation to submit a story at a *different* site followed the "We are not currently accepting births stories" sentence. *Childbirth.org* offers only the illusion of inviting women to share. The message remains an odd mix of invitation and denial; still not itself accepting stories but with ever-updated "ads by Google" on the page, the site treats women as consumers but not as contributors.

By contrast, the 2005 iteration of *TheLaborofLove.com* was straightforward and apologetic about its hiatus from accepting and posting new stories. The note "We're sorry, but at this time, we are not accepting new birth stories" appeared on the birth stories index page. This note, however, was nearly buried at the bottom of a busy page, most of which was taken up with graphic and text advertisements for everything from 4-D ultrasound to medical insurance, demonstrating that, like at *Childbirth.org*, at *TheLaborofLove.com* the desire to sell was stronger than the desire to give women a voice.

By 2010, *TheLaborofLove.com* included a "Submit Birth Story" button on the birth stories section of the site, but access to that site was complicated and the process saturated with targeted advertisements. To submit a story a reader would first register and see above the registration/login space the image from the *Business of Being Born* (2008) poster and DVD. A reader clicking on a birth story would also see that same image: no story was without an accompanying *Business of Being Born* image and log-in option, suggesting a continuous sponsorship. Within the birth stories themselves, particular words like "baby" or "pregnancy" are hyperlinked; clicking those links reveals commercials for items like First Response (a pregnancy test).

During its hiatus from accepting new stories, *TheLaborofLove.com* seems to have identified new ways to capitalize on women's words and new ways to control their stories. For example, the site's invitation to write, a form that women fill out online, asks writers to choose only one of thirteen categories, essentially asking women to privilege one aspect of their childbirth experience over another (such as type of intervention over number birth). The form also asks for an "Author Alias" but not the author's actual name. The form does, however, provide an open space in which writers may type and offers writers authorial control over when the story will go live and when it will go offline.

These categorizations and invitations to write illustrate one way in which the genre of the online birth story is remediated and differs from earlier iterations of written birth stories. This is not to suggest that, for example, Victorian women writing birth stories in letters did not have any constraints on their language choices, for certainly they did, but those women were not being guided or encouraged to use specific labels that would bring consumer traffic. Such inventional direction and improvisational constraint suggest a distinction between the genre of the online birth story, particularly at the corporate sites, and other birth story genres.

The noncorporate sites also guide stories, though in different ways. *Plomp.com* simply asks women to send in their stories, while *UnassistedChildbirth.com*, by contrast, is quite prescriptive. Even the placement of the invitation to write at *UnassistedChildbirth.com* suggests the expectation of immersion in the philosophy of the site. The request to submit birth stories is embedded within an invitation to join an online unassisted childbirth forum; the stories on this site do not belong to women who happen to see a "share your story!" suggestion. The women writing for this site hold particular beliefs or have particular experiences that led them to seek out this site. These beliefs encompass not only birth but also these women's places in the world.

As the site title would suggest, *UnassistedChildbirth.com* deals exclusively with a specific type of home birth, an "unassisted" birth where women opt to have not only no physician present but no midwife, no doula, often no one at all. The only exception to the unassisted birth story on the site is when some women frame their unassisted birth with an earlier experience of a hospital or birth center birth; these births are presented in stark contrast to, and always as foils against, their later triumphant, unassisted home births. One mother's concluding sentence sums up an assertion many mothers on *UnassistedChildbirth.com* make: "It was birth the way it should be: an ordinary miracle" (Laurie, "Ordinary Miracle"). On this site the viewpoint is that birth is the woman's domain—not *women*'s, but the birthing woman alone.

UnassistedChildbirth.com is the only site of the five examined to have explicit expectations, or litmus tests, for the type of stories posted, but unlike at the corporate sites, the constraints here have no consumer-focused end in mind. Rather, the site could be seen as anticonsumerist. A few stories at the site describe accidental unassisted home births, which often end with a declaration that all births should be this way. Kym, for example, who had planned a birth center birth, instead had an accidental home birth—with surprise twins!—and concludes that she "cannot imagine having gone to the hospital or even the birth center after such beautiful births" ("Home Sweet Home Home"). *UnassistedChildbirth.com* provides a forum for women with birth stories far outside the American mainstream to safely share their stories of successfully asserting feminist agency over their births. At this site they can challenge the dominant cultural script for childbirth in the United States and expect support for their childbirth beliefs.

CONCLUDING BY WAY OF IMAGES

As the explorations above have illustrated, each website provides readers access to particular notions of childbirth. While the corporate sites all tend to fit with current dominant childbirth norms (including the norm of a certain degree of resistance to childbirth norms), focusing particularly on consumer needs, the noncorporate sites offer less consumer-focused alternatives. While the sites' copyright policies, categorizations, invitations to write, and the women's stories themselves provide a variety of ways for readers to assess a site's match with their own beliefs and developing orientations to childbirth, images on the sites may most readily demonstrate the particular audience the site intends to reach, the community it intends to create or sustain, and the belief systems it reflects or advances.

The look of a given site allows readers to immediately self-select based on what appeals to them. Most of the sites, such as *TheLaborofLove.com*, provide images of babies, teddy bears, and parent/child, hand/foot contrasts, images that focus on clean babies and an impersonal culture of "cute" as opposed to writers' own images of childbirth itself. Personal images are not typically present at any of the corporate sites, but both Plomp and Shanley invite readers to send in photographs with their stories. The women who choose this option tend to include pictures of the baby clothed in a favorite outfit or pictures of mom and baby well after the birth, rather than a photo documenting the birth itself. Plomp's own photograph is the most graphic on the site, a torso shot of herself gazing at her daughter shortly after the birth; while she is topless, her baby covers her nipples and the lower half of her breasts (Plomp, "Birth Story of Tamara").

At *UnassistedChildbirth.com*, by contrast, pictures are significantly less demure (Fig. 4.1). The images on this site glory in the changed pregnant form and the birthing body. There is no dearth of naked birth pictures, and a section of the site is devoted to birth erotica. Images of fully nude women breast-feeding are not uncommon. Many of the images tend to eroticize and/or romanticize the pregnant female figure. Figure 4.1 illustrates the image styles on this site. Images accompanying several stories echo the soft-focus, black-and-white nude profile of a very pregnant woman gazing at a long-stemmed rose.

Carol Stabile points out that in popular American culture, "the pregnant body—even clothed—is a source of abjection and disgust . . . the woman is represented as awkward, uncomfortable, and grotesquely excessive" (183). The images on *UnassistedChildbirth.com* defy this popular—though possibly outdated—conception, instead celebrating the pregnant form. In doing so they disrupt expectations, similar to the way that Annie Leibovitz's cover shot of Demi Moore did in the August 1991 issue of *Vanity Fair.* As Barbara Dickson notes in her essay analyzing that image, "to display the pregnant body as sexually desirable undoes conventionality" (301). Although the birth pictures are snapshots, taken by partners or friends,[9] many of the pregnancy photographs, like that *Vanity Fair* image, are professional photographs. These women's beliefs about their bodies and their places in

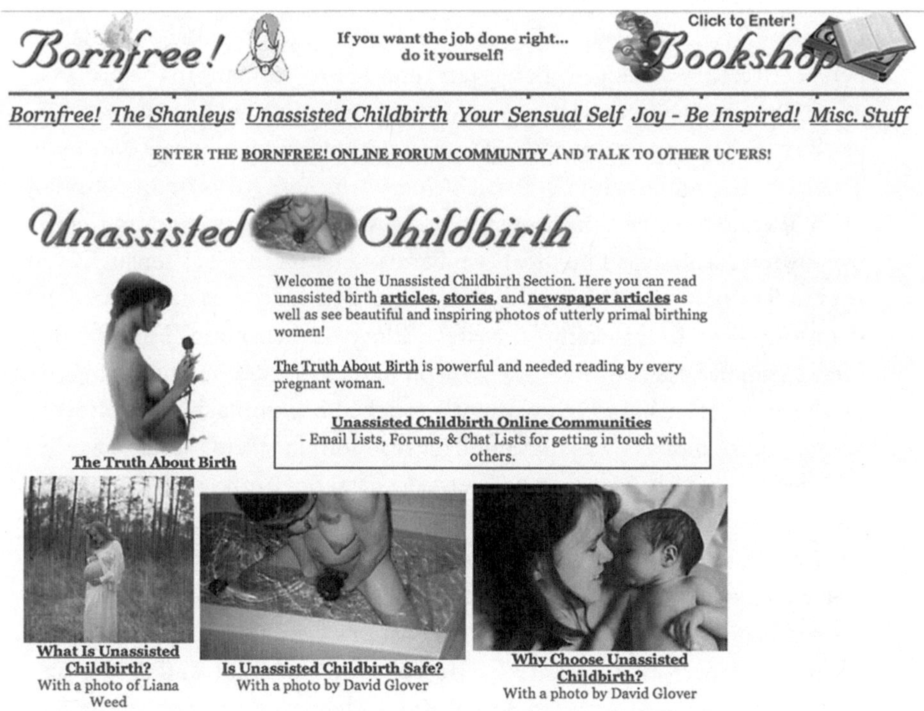

Figure 4.1. Birth and pregnancy images. *Courtesy of Laura Kaplan Shanley, author of* Unassisted Childbirth

society manifest themselves not only in their choices to birth unassisted at home and to share the stories of these births online but also in their hiring of photographers to document their changing bodies in particularly staged ways. By sharing these images on the websites alongside their stories, these women make public their beliefs, remediate their pregnancies, challenge societal expectations, and encourage other women to do so as well.

Images serve as a striking example of the distinction between *UnassistedChildbirth.com* as a specialized birthing site and the corporate sites as more general birthing sites. None of the three corporate sites offer readers the option of sending photographs to accompany stories (although the site to which *Childbirth.org* was sending prospective writers by 2010, *Pregnancy.about.com*, does provide that option). For years, however, *Childbirth.org* linked to a page offering pictures of "pregnant bellies" sent in by readers. The pictures were organized by number of weeks pregnant and offered images usually of fully clothed women (often in sweatpants) standing in profile and lifting their shirts to reveal their changed/changing stomachs. Several of the pictures were cropped so women were decapitated and seemed to have no lower legs. These images, literally just bellies, had no erotic or romantic perspective; they cataloged change (and erased the "woman" in the process).

Of the five sites in this study, only *UnassistedChildbirth.com* seems interested in presenting a view of the pregnant or birthing woman *as a woman*. These images, along with *UnassistedChildbirth.com*'s focus on one kind of birth, dictate the style and content of stories. Nearly every story on the site overtly rejects birth as a medical event and often presents it as sensual, even sexy, a feminist recasting of the dominant, decidedly unsensual medical definition. Karen, for example, writes, "I love the sensations I am having. They mean baby is coming!" She goes on to describe a moment during her birth when her husband inadvertently touched her stomach in an effort to see what progress she was making. Her reaction illustrates her conception of labor as something a woman must do herself: "I immediately lost my concentration, and yelled at him 'Hey! Get your hand out of there! You are worse than an OB!' and I spanked him pretty hard on his butt." Karen freely challenges the widely accepted belief in the United States that birth is a medical event best attended by an obstetrician. She further challenges common modern expectations that husbands/partners can and should play a hands-on role in labor and delivery. Karen shares her story at *UnassistedChildbirth.com* for a community predisposed to accept it—where rejection of dominant childbirth conventions *is* the convention.

UnassistedChildbirth.com provides a safe haven for nonconventional birthers to read and share birth information, including images, and both the stories and site consistently reflect that expectation. By resisting cultural norms that give authority over birth to trained professionals, the site instead adheres to norms of antiestablishment, a view made visible through content, links, and images on the site. But this site, although unique in this study for its targeted focus and use of images and with its promise of shared beliefs and knowledge, is not different from the other four sites in that it makes no active move to connect women to each other.

None of these sites permits readers to comment on or otherwise interact with the stories. Although I have argued that the sites seek to provide some sense of virtual coterie for women in something of a reinterpretation of the historical trend of "social childbirth," I have also made clear that the sites fail more often than they succeed in this regard. And although this study does not include Web 2.0 spaces, it seems incumbent to mention briefly that the spaces typically provided for comments in those environments would also be unlikely to virtually recreate a social childbirth scene akin to that of colonial times in North America. Such extant nonrestricted spaces, with their allowance for comments from disparate types of distant Facebook friends or often-anonymous blog visitors, are unlikely to yield a supportive birthing coterie.

And yet the possibility for emotional, psychological, and physical benefits from social networking sites does exist and is beginning to be explored (see, for example, Santos). Writing and posting a birth story may not create a productive virtual birth coterie, and online spaces may not consistently enhance women's rhetorical agency, but yet, as the next chapter will demonstrate, the act of writing and posting an online birth story does, for the women in this study, seem to have beneficial emotional, psychological, and even physical effects. The next chapter digs into women's online birth stories and survey responses to illuminate the cathartic effects of their writing, the variety and significance of their rhetorical stances, and the ways women use their online birth stories to retroactively claim agency over their births.

CHAPTER FIVE

SHARiNG BiRTH

Catharsis, Commentary, and Testimonial in Online Birth Stories

> Individuals have the capacity to call upon . . . multiple influences to fashion rhetorics of their own, creating personal and collective narratives of history and experiences that can disrupt the interests of dominant institutions.
>
> —John Duffy, "Other Gods and Countries"

Childbirth is a profoundly significant, transformative event—not only physically but psychologically and socially as well. It can be cathartic, in the sense of "linking of thoughts and feelings" (Pennebaker 39) and in each sense of the three distinct definitions of catharsis the online *Oxford English Dictionary* provides:

a. Purgation of the excrements of the body; esp. evacuation of the bowels.
b. The purification of the emotions by vicarious experience, esp. through the drama (in reference to Aristotle's Poetics 6). Also more widely.
c. Psychotherapy. The process of relieving an abnormal excitement by re-establishing the association of the emotion with the memory or idea of the event which was the first cause of it, and of eliminating it by abreaction. ("Catharsis")

While childbirth is potentially cathartic in a physical and metaphysical sense, childbirth writing, too, is also potentially cathartic in a metaphysical sense, though sometimes with bodily implications, as in the release of stress. Psychologists and writing scholars alike have found that writing can provide or encourage catharsis for the writer (see, for example, Pennebaker; Harris).

Online birth narratives often demonstrate catharsis both implicitly and explicitly. As chapter 3 demonstrated, birthing women can be perceived as (and feel) unstable, or rhetorically disabled. Writing birth narratives may restore women's voices, enabling them to impose rhetorical agency after the fact, as mothers and as mindful, healthy people; we might call them "rhetorically enabled subjects," to borrow Catherine Prendergast's phrase (200). Oral narratives may also serve this purpose to a certain extent, but as Judith Harris, author of *Signifying Pain*, argues, writing "permits the careful construction of a cohesive narrative in a way that simply talking about experiences does not" (56).[1] The act of writing encourages, or permits, both catharsis and self-analysis.

This chapter shows that these cathartic and self-analytical elements of writing apply to online birth narratives and demonstrates that many women use the narratives of their experience as a form of sociopolitical expression. The chapter also shows how women's consumer identities filter through the narratives. Further, it argues that online birth stories reflect and challenge theoretical understandings of narrative and memory.

As John Duffy explains in "Other Gods and Countries," people create their own narratives of experiences; these narratives, in the form of women's online birth narratives, have a disruptive potential that works in two ways. First, the stories (can) disrupt women's own memories of their births, a disruption that has the potential to affect the way they continue on in their roles as mothers, as patients, and as participants in a larger society. Second, these stories posted on publicly accessible websites enable other women to see birth (as well as societal roles as women and as mothers) through the writers' eyes, which can disrupt other women's expectations of childbirth, disrupt the dominant cultural scripts for childbirth (see chapter 1), and disrupt both readers' birth plans (written documents) and their plans for birth (decisions about where and with whose assistance they will give birth). Each of these disruptions can, in turn and in time, affect the dominant institutions of childbirth, even if they do not successfully affect an individual writer's experience giving birth.

Feminist rhetorical agency distributed across time and space can produce lasting effects, as we saw in chapter 2 with the changes to routine enemas. If women's choices increasingly reflect desires for change, change will come. Birth stories like the ones in this study could contribute to such change, and yet for the story authors in my study, their most memorable comments about the effects of writing their stories had to do with the change in themselves.

The women I surveyed claimed repeatedly and forcefully that writing online birth stories was cathartic for them. Composing childbirth narratives allows women the opportunity to relive the bodily experience of birth emotionally and psychologically, often allowing them to reassert rhetorical agency over their births in doing so. The writing mimics, to a certain extent, the event itself, but in this reproduction, this remediation, the woman herself—rather than her body, birth attendants, or technology—controls every aspect of the story. This retroactive assertion of agency may be one reason women find writing birth narratives to be cathartic.

CATHARSIS AND SOCIOPOLITICAL EXPRESSION

In women's online birth narratives, the personal is often implicitly political, reflecting that credo of second-wave feminism. These stories are also often rather overtly political: for example, women advocate particular stances and childbirth choices that have subtle but significant social and political ramifications. This writing follows a somewhat hidden history of women's writing; as Kathryn Flannery has shown, women's writing, albeit essential in obtaining feminist advances, has often been discounted or ignored in mainstream histories. Even women's writing intended as public has been deemed private.

While birth story authors may seem to be simply sharing personal stories, they also use this form of public writing to advance political and social goals. Gail Hawisher and Patricia Sullivan claim that even though women may not always know how to "harness e-spaces as sites for feminist power . . . women's participation in e-space will necessitate a rethinking of public and private space" (195). Women writing online birth stories, like other women in the general public, may not identify themselves as "feminists"—indeed, my survey participants did not typically identify as such—but their actions nonetheless demonstrate their ability to harness e-spaces for causes I would call feminist.[2] My analysis of these online birth narratives both highlights the integration of the personal and the political so common in this genre and complicates how we understand or categorize women's writing.

Women's birth narratives are useful not only for the women who write them; indeed, they are consistently produced and read as educational tools for other women, some with an eye toward explicitly challenging dominant beliefs about childbirth. These narratives can function, then, both as personal writing and as political writing. The catharsis enabled by such writing helps women themselves but also works to help and educate other women, both covertly through personal stories—where personal experience serves as warrant for a larger political claim—and overtly through particular recommendations and advice.

I asked survey respondents to complete the following sentence: "Writing/ posting this story was _____ for me." Responses seemed to coalesce into emotional categories; I identified three: complex, positive, and transformative. Ambiguous emotional responses that were neither clearly positive nor transformative, such as "sentimental" and "scary," I labeled "complex." I called "transformative" any term that denoted a change from one emotional state to another, such as "healing, "therapeutic," or "cathartic." Words like "exciting" and "enjoyable" did not seem to connote a perceptive shift and were placed into the more static "positive" category. Thirty-one women answered this question, sometimes giving multiple responses that I coded differently, so the percentages add up to more than 100. Six responses, or 19 percent, were complex; eleven, or 35 percent, were positive, while sixteen, or 52 percent, fell into the transformative category.[3] For more than half of these women, then, writing the birth story produced a significant emotional change.

Another question, "What effect did you intend your story to have on others? On yourself?" also revealed cathartic results for women. Many women wrote of emotional transformations or other benefits they experienced through writing:

> It was like therapy to write it. (slimgirl156, survey)
>
> It was good for me to write it down when I did. (Katrina, survey)
>
> It was just something that affected me deeply and needed to be written down to stop bothering me so much. (Anna, survey)
>
> It was therapeutic for me to be able to go back over the events of my experience. (Shannon, survey)
>
> I thought that writing down my experience to help others would make me feel better about the things I did not like in my birth experience. (Beth, survey)

> When I write something down I am more easily able to let it go, and I don't sit and dwell on it as much. (Michele, survey)

> To empower myself. (Autumn, survey)

While a few women had more simple, casual expectations such as "It was fun" (Julie, survey) or wrote "to satisfy [other pregnant women's] curiosity" (Anna, survey), the majority of responses extends the idea that writing the birth story provided an emotional release. Responses here further establish the cathartic value of posting birth stories for many of these women. They also hint at the significant issues of memory and the (re)construction of experiences through narrative, which will be explored later in this chapter.

For these women, writing birth stories served a powerful transformative purpose. The majority of them set out to write their stories with an eye toward helping themselves emotionally. They used writing to (re)mediate their experiences and overcame what sociologist Ann Oakley calls "victim" status in doing so. Oakley's determination of victim versus victor status relies upon a woman's social network, the level of medical intervention in the birth, and how the mother deals with her emotions about the medicalization. Oakley's categorization of postpartum women relies on women's *interpretations* of the birth as much as it does on the facts or experience of the birth. Readers might expect traumatic births to provide fodder for cathartic writing, and this is indeed the case in the sense that seven of the sixteen women who experienced catharsis through writing had births that did not go as planned, births where interventions and/or complications deviated drastically from their expectations. However, even some women who had an almost ideal childbirth wrote of experiencing catharsis through writing birth narratives. Five of the sixteen women in the transformative category described births that went extremely well—both by medical and their own emotional standards.[4] This finding suggests that writing provides an emotional release not only for those who feel traumatized by their births but also for births across the wide continuum of experiences.

CONSUMER TESTIMONIALS: ADVICE IN BIRTH NARRATIVES

This study reveals two additional, interrelated purposes for women writing online birth narratives, beyond writing for personal catharsis or sociopolitical expression: to provide commentary on services rendered—a sort of birth consumer testimonial, complete with product or service recommendations—and to solicit responses to their stories for emotional or informational exchange. Some women encourage readers to contact them, seeking to forge connections that might help both themselves and others. As discussed in chapter 4, though, the connective promise of the web is often unfulfilled. But while the anticipated exchange may not be achieved, the rhetorical choice to permit or invite that connection is significant for the authors. Women in the survey often express their hope that others would respond to their stories. Carolyn offers a poignant example: "My birth did not go as planned and I wanted to be reassured that it was not my fault" (survey).

The online narratives also reveal women's beliefs about the connective power of the Internet. Two women in particular who end their stories with explicit advice alongside invitations to write to them are Jenny and Beth. (Readers have already been introduced to Beth, whose birth plan and survey data appear in chapter 3.) Jenny writes: "Well, there's my story. I would be happy to share more information on hospital birth, c-section, homebirth, postpartum depression with anyone interested. Jenny [link to her email address]." Beth closes her narrative with the following: "Here is my advice for all expecting mothers—(1) read all the birth stories you can, and (2) make a birth plan so others will know what you want when you can't speak for yourself. If you have any questions or have had a similar experience and would like to contact me please feel free to do so. My email address is . . ." Jenny and Beth both offer readers the opportunity to connect with them. They see the birth story as a valuable source of information for others. Beth encourages women to inform themselves and almost to arm themselves. Both writers' advice suggests that women need to protect themselves from birth practices, a political position aimed at helping other women.

Those I surveyed explicitly acknowledged hopes that their writing would help other women. Other responses to the question "What effect did you intend your story to have on others?" yielded responses that demonstrate this belief:

> I intended the effect of my stories to be one of a positive nature towards the practice of natural and unmedicated childbirth. (Shannon, survey)

> I hoped my stories would encourage women to look at all options in childbirth. (Jessica, survey)

> I . . . want to share positive homebirth stories to encourage women to look at safe options for childbirth. (Sherry, survey)
>
> Maybe it would make them [other pregnant women] realize that it is possible to give birth out of the hospital, and be ok. (Karen, survey)
>
> I wanted other pregnant women to know that even with a complicated pregnancy, the outcome can still be a positive one. (Melissa, survey)
>
> To share, to teach. (Jennifer, survey)

Each of these women offers her story, then, not simply out of a desire for personal benefit but to persuade, teach, or otherwise inspire her audience.

Birth narratives function not only as personal records and sociopolitical commentaries but also as product or service testimonials. Women testify in their stories that particular services are worthwhile, particular types of attendants helpful, particular locations better than others. In providing these service recommendations, women display themselves as satisfied (or dissatisfied) customers. This consumer element adds another layer to the competing interests and influences at play in this genre. As we see in the above comment by Karen, who wants readers to "realize that it is possible to give birth out of the hospital, and be ok," some women write out of a conscious desire to affect other women's opinions and increase their knowledge. The expressivist bent of the birth narrative is superseded by a transactional desire to persuade readers that reading or writing such narratives can transform and improve other women's birth experiences.

Survey respondents reflected, as asked, on their completed birth narratives and provided metadata about their intentions while writing, but the narratives themselves also reveal these impulses. Online birth stories share all things personal—intimate details about everything from sex in labor to gory surgeries—but many reveal an explicit dual purpose by the end of the narrative. The birth finished, the baby born, reactions registered, the stories become part advice column, part consciousness-raising tract. Sherry provides one example of this rhetorical move, beginning by explaining the day, date, and how far along she was and continuing to describe her laboring hours with an inward focus, following the expected conventions of the genre. In her final paragraph, however, she shifts attention to the reader:

> For more information on natural childbirth, I recommend reading the following books: *Birth Reborn* by Michel Odent, M.D., *Childbirth Without Fear* by Dr. Grantly Dick-Read, *Husband-Coached Childbirth* by Dr. Robert Bradley and *Birthrights* by Sally Inch. I read more than twenty pregnancy-related books during this pregnancy, but these are some of my favorites *having information that you may not be able to find anywhere else.* (my emphasis)

The significance of Sherry's rhetorical move away from describing her experience and toward offering advice extends beyond her awareness of her audience as women seeking knowledge about the birth process. This move speaks to her belief that even the wealth of information about childbirth—offered by doctors, in childbirth classes, and in countless books combined—is not always complete. Sherry is "convinced that home birth with [only] intermittent fetal monitoring and someone trained to deal with complications is the safest way to have a baby," a view that resists dominant understandings and institutions in American society. She uses her writing to document her own resistance and to encourage other women to question widespread assumptions, to educate themselves against the common grain.

Recommendations do not always work against the traditional American hospital birth experience, though; some women suggest epidurals, particular painkillers, even C-sections. What the recommendations all have in common, however, is their function as consumer testimonials. These testimonials are sometimes overtly aimed at an audience but can also be couched in terms of personal preference, with the preferences shared in such a way that they operate as recommendations.

> I would suggest to anyone having a c-section to write a birth plan. (Melissa, survey)

> Anyway, my advice to pregnant women is this: epidural! and breathe. (Krystle, survey)

> If you're trying to figure out which birthing method to try, check out birth hypnosis! It works! (Summer, survey)

> I would never have a baby any other place than at home, and I would never suggest anything else for anyone. (Autumn, survey)

> Good luck to all the mothers-to-be who read this. And do not let others tell you that what you are doing during pregnancy is wrong. Just because those who are going through it or have been through it weren't able to, doesn't mean that it does apply to you. (Jess, survey)

> In response to the recent concerns surrounding VBAC (Vaginal Birth After Cesarean) I wanted to write my birth story and give hope to those wanting to experience a vaginal delivery after a cesarean. . . . Take Care and God Bless. (Amy, survey)

> I am also glad we hired the doula, she was great and I wouldn't have been able to go natural without her I know it. . . . I'm also glad that I did a lot of research and knew my rights and my desires for my birth. (Cynthia, survey)

Where Melissa and Krystle simply offer their recommendations, Summer and Autumn both connect their advice to their own experiences. Readers are left to believe that because hypnosis worked for Summer, it could, and even should, for them. Autumn's preference for a home birth may be a hard sell in the United States with its presumption of hospital births, but her rhetorical impulse is the same as Summer's: the personal is the political; one story could be everywoman's story. Jess, however, complicates this strategy through her advice that other women's (bad) experiences should not be a reason not to do or try something. Jess seems to be writing against the prototypical "horror story" (see chapter 4).

Women often tell their own tales of thwarted expectations and in doing so imply to other women that their hopes—for a drug-free labor, for any particular or positive birth experience—are unreachable. Jess, then, hints at an understanding that all women's experiences are different, at least in terms of ignoring negative stories. Amy writes to offer, simply, "hope," using her experience as the proof that such hope is warranted. Cynthia's declaration that she felt capable of natural birth only because she had a doula serves as a powerful suggestion to other women that they, too, can benefit from a doula. In asserting her own experience, Cynthia makes the implicit claim that if other women make the same choices and do their homework (in her terms, "a lot of research"), they too can get the birth they want. (Her assertion may not hold true for everyone, though, as we see for the five women in chapter 3.) Each of these women writes to support and influence other women's choices as consumers.

It is important to bear in mind that women have historically acted as *consumers* of childbirth services. Online birth narratives are not the first instance in history of women advocating particular consumer choices: recall that women *invited* physicians to their birthing rooms and, in an early feminist bid, argued for their rights to hospital births and anesthetized birth (see Leavitt, particularly on twilight sleep, *Brought to Bed* 128–40). While early twentieth-century American women's fight for the right to obstetric interventions and access to hospital admission was relatively easily won, later efforts (by some) to avoid obstetric interventions in an era where hospital admission for childbirth is nearly universal have been much more fraught. The changes in childbirth—perhaps most notably in the locus of control surrounding childbirth, once firmly within the birthing woman's sphere, now firmly in the birth attendant's sphere—may suggest that becoming a particular kind of consumer produces lasting change, change that may not always prove beneficial to women.

Women's expectations as consumers have shaped their political goals and accomplishments, but those political accomplishments have, in turn, shaped women's expectations as consumers. With regard to childbirth, such consumer expectations are layered with the emotional and sociopolitical significance of both childbirth itself and of childbirth writing. While women's identities as consumers do not replace their other crucial identities, the childbirth narratives offer a palimpsest of these various identities. The consumer testimonial and the traditional birth narrative merge, particularly in this online environment, to form a new genre. This new genre reflects pregnant/birthing American women's response to being treated and constructed by others as consumers first and anything else second. (For more on consumerism and motherhood, specifically, see Taylor, Layne, and Wozniak.)

"*MY* EPIDURAL": RHETORICAL CONSTRUCTIONS OF CONSUMER ENTITLEMENT

> Jay told me that at this stage I was still begging for an epidural and everyone had just given up and kept telling me the anaesthetist was on his way. Now my dad told me his most memorable moment was me screaming "Can't you people f****ing hear me? I want my f****ing

> epidural—wheres my f****ing epidural???" (the only time i swore during the whole entire event). (Danielle)

Women's expectations as consumers are reflected in the narratives in constructions such as "my epidural," suggestive of a certain sense of consumer entitlement as well as rhetorical agency. This phrasing is particularly poignant when women write about the epidural in the possessive before they have one or even when they never get one. Women's epidural expectations are often thwarted by anything from the particulars of birth experiences to hospital staffing to medication simply not "taking." Any deviation from expectations can produce a dissatisfied customer. Online narratives offer a range of consumer responses:

> Not too long after I was admitted, I was given my epidural. What a life saver! I was able to relax and call people to tell them I was in labor. (Kim)

> I was really happy when they came to get me because I knew I'd get my epidural in a matter of minutes. I was having a c-section, I wasn't supposed to feel any pain until afterwords! I was taken to the OR and got my epidural. (Melissa)

> I got my epidural, but barely. If they hadn't checked me, it would've been too late. (Krystle)

> We arrived at the hospital at 14:50 and I promptly and politely started requesting my epidural. I was taken to a labour room and left for 20 minutes. . . . I was told the anaesthetist was elsewhere and would be with us as soon as he could. What! I wanted my epidural and I wanted it now! She said she had better put down that I was 5cm dilated because any more and I wouldn't get my epidural (I was actually 6cm). . . . At 15:30 I was told the anaesthetist would be half an hour. Panic set in because things were going so fast, . . . and I hadn't had my epidural. (Thomas's mother)

Kim's description of her epidural follows a standard rhetorical pattern for testimonials: she states the intervention received and describes its benefits. Melissa's narrative, too, reflects this pattern; beyond this, however, she includes the expectation that she feel *no* pain. Her phrasing notes the potential for dissatisfaction ("I wasn't supposed to feel any pain") and suggests that as a customer, she was satisfied, but only barely. Krystle shares a similar story, hinting that the nameless "they" almost made an egregious error of timing. Thomas's mother offers perhaps the most interesting use of the possessive because the epidural she repeatedly refers to as hers is one she never receives, despite her hopes and the nurse's willing collusion to permit her one after the time typically deemed appropriate.

By writing of particular medical services in the possessive, these women construct themselves as entitled consumers, as patients with rights, as women with rhetorical agency over the medical pain assistance they expect to have with their births. These narratives represent a common thread in online birth narratives of women writing as consumers. These remediations of childbirth reflect the multiple lenses through which women review their births: personal experience, sociopolitical significance, and consumer influence.

RHETORICAL STANCE FORMATION IN BIRTH NARRATIVES

As we saw with the women who wrote of even nonexistent epidurals in the possessive, consumer expectations affect women's stances toward their births, not only as the birth events unfold but in their construction of the experience afterward. Women's narratives often display multiple and often somewhat contradictory positions that ultimately coalesce into a stable rhetorical stance. That women occupy different and contradictory positions provides an example of Karlyn Kohrs Campbell's explanation that "culturally available subject-positions are, simultaneously, obstacles and opportunities, but they are shifting, not fixed, identities" (4). Women take on different roles, even within a single birth narrative, and one way we see these personae reflected is in the interplay of passive voice and active voice. Passive voice, for example, may be a rhetorical and grammatical reflection of a somewhat passive acceptance of American birth practices. Active voice, on the other hand, may reflect a desire for agency, which for some suggests resistance to particular birth practices or of hospital hierarchies, more generally. Most narratives offer a mixture of the passive and the active, a blend of distinct subject positions held by a single woman in a single narrative. This complexity mirrors the complexity of birth itself as a profound physical, psychological, social, and often medical event.

Readers might expect hospital birth narratives to reflect passivity and home-birth narratives to reflect significant agency. Based on the narratives included in my study, I find that for home births, this expectation generally holds true. For hospital births, however, by far the majority, the results are much less easily delineated. Particular stances are most visible when formed against a norm; the most poignant examples, then, arise from those women whose writing offers some challenge to accepted practices. To illustrate the variety of rhetorical stances, I quote extensively from two hospital birth narratives, those of Sandy and Jennifer, teasing out the rhetorical stances each comes to in turn.

ACCEPTANCE AND RESISTANCE: SANDY AND JENNIFER

One birth narrative, Sandy's, demonstrates a shift from disappointment, potential dissatisfaction, and attempts at agency to complete acceptance. This shift is marked, in part, by her increasing dependence upon the passive voice to tell her story. Her story opens with her quest to become pregnant—an eight-year process—and leads into her demonstration of her educational knowledge about childbirth, an indication of agency: "I had read every book and article I could find on everything about childbirth and labor and what to expect." Upon describing her arrival at the hospital, however, she begins to rely on the passive voice. Her story becomes less the story of her son's birth and more the story of what was done to/for/around her:

> I was met at the emergency room door . . . I was left in the emergency room waiting . . . I was finally retrieved and taken to the Maternity floor . . . I was told to go to the bathroom (for the last time) and slip into my gown. I was then put in bed and hooked up to a monitor. I didn't like that because I wanted to walk around. They told me I couldn't because of the risk of an infection. . . . We had talked in general during my visits about Cesarean, and I had expressed to him that I surely didn't want one of those. However, since they couldn't get a good reading on the baby (they kept losing his heart beat on the monitor and I was still only 1 cm after 7 hours), they had to do one. I was clearly upset. However, Dr. Duff and the nurses reassured me and kept me calm . . . a catheter was put in . . . I was given a shot . . . I was kept in recovery for 4 hours due to my low blood pressure, but Zachary was brought in and I was allowed to hold him and nurse him for the first time.

From her entrance in the hospital, Sandy describes things that happen almost as if she were not present. She was met, left, retrieved, taken, told, put in bed, and hooked to a monitor. At this point in the narrative, although the passive voice is overwhelming, Sandy's sense of her own agency has not disappeared, however. Having read numerous books and articles about childbirth and what to expect, she initially expresses her reluctance to being hooked up to a monitor. She writes of her dissatisfaction, of her thwarted desire to walk during labor.[5] Told that a C-section "had" to be performed, her emotions momentarily take center stage; her agency becomes apparent in her wish to avoid this operation. Quickly calmed, however, Sandy writes again with a string of passive constructions: a catheter was put in and she was given a shot, was kept in recovery, and was allowed to hold and nurse her son.

Sandy's narrative does not seek to empower other women or to challenge any beliefs about childbirth. Her narrative operates in the usual sense of narrative: to reaffirm established norms of acceptance and compliance. Her story (re)mediates her birth experience in that it helps her reconcile her expectations for birth with her very different experiences. For Sandy, acceptance of the birth experience comes in part through writing about it. Even while she may seem to lack agency, both in her birth experience and in her writing of it, Sandy's narrative serves as an example of how online childbirth writing permits transcendence: a move from disappointment to acceptance. Her writing enables the formation of this accepting rhetorical stance.

Jennifer's narrative stands in stark contrast to Sandy's. While it accomplishes similar personal goals in that it permits transcendence and helps her reconcile expectations with experiences, she often positions herself in roles of active resistance. Passive constructions are nearly absent from her story, but even so her resistance wavers. Like Sandy, although on the opposite end of the spectrum, her writing persona is not always consistent but nonetheless coalesces into a stable rhetorical stance.

> We discussed putting in an internal contraction monitor so they could officially tell me that my occasional dinky contractions weren't doing anything. Of course during our discussion he failed to provide full informed consent, neglecting to tell me that I would not be able to get out of bed with it in. . . . I told everyone I was going to the shower unhooked my monitor and went. . . . Within moments I could feel her crown, and reached my hand down to support my perinium. I caught her head in my hands. I said that her head was out and a nurse walking into the room yelled down the hall for the OB (damn her, I was doing fine). I flipped over and pushed her the rest of the way out right when the OB arrived

> . . . the doctor . . . started tugging on my cord to get the placenta. I told him to stop, but he said it was almost out anyway. . . . Several days after [my daughter] was born I developed a uterine infection from small pieces of retained placenta, due to it having been pulled out. Overall I had a good birth, but I am disappointed with the way the doctor treated us. Next time will definatly be at home.

Jennifer's narrative does little to support norms. Her retrospective story, instead, repeatedly resists norms. She writes of the decision to have "official" notification that her contractions were not progressing her labor, but her rhetorical construction suggests she already knew this: here Jennifer's narrative offers a conflicting positioning, one of simultaneous trust in her own bodily knowledge even as she accepts a technological reading of the same situation. Both her writing and her actions reflect these contradictory positions: for example, she accepts an internal monitor that keeps her in bed but then unhooks it herself to take a shower.

Moments of Jennifer's agency and resistance in the narrative are interspersed with episodes of somewhat passive acceptance. This is apparent in her description of the actual birth. She constructs her description to reveal herself as the sole agent in her early delivery: she provides her own perineal support, catches the baby's head, and announces her progress to a nurse (who then calls for the doctor). Jennifer's interjection into her own story—"(damn her, I was doing fine)"—suggests her feeling that her empowerment was thwarted or at least challenged by the nurse's reaction. She describes the third stage of labor as almost a retaliation story, as if the doctor pulled her placenta out to prove that he had done something, since she delivered the baby herself. Her infection is described as a direct result of his unwanted actions, serving in the narrative as both moral (she knew best) and retaliation. Her narrative reveals a rhetorical stance in which she accepts her birth experience without accepting her physician's treatment choices; Jennifer writes herself into a place where she can take responsibility for the aspects of the experience she did not like. She accepts this because she chose to place herself in the hospital. She also demonstrates agency in her final statement, that her next birth will be a home birth. Implicit in this statement is the belief that in her home she will be able to exert more control.

Sandy and Jennifer both arrive at rhetorical stances that are more complex than Oakley's victim/victor binary would allow for; each woman writes from multiple positions, as if casting about for the appropriate place to land.

The rhetorical stances they land on serve their individual purposes, freeing each from difficult memories. These two narratives provide extended examples of how two women come to productive rhetorical stances, but these are, of course, not exhaustive.

Other women write of their contentedness with hospital protocols. Anna, for example, found comfort in being "safely strapped in [her] hospital bed with the baby monitor." While other women find such straps limiting to movement and agency, Anna speaks for those who gratefully accept such routines. Anna writes calmly and seemingly without curiosity that after she gave birth to her daughter, "her daddy cut her cord and they took her (and her daddy) into the next room to do whatever they do to newborns." While many women want immediate and constant access to their newborns, despite hospital routines that often separate them, Anna finds no such conflict. She writes from a place of acceptance, but unlike for Sandy or Jennifer, this acceptance does not seem fraught; instead it seems to come easily, whether as a result of her birth, her personality, or something else that is not apparent. Her stance, then, is one of contented trust.

Trust and acceptance contrast, of course, with distrust and sometimes anger. Women who write of more than one birth experience necessarily create a stance toward earlier births that refracts through later birth experiences; when women write of hospital births that preceded home births, this contrast is particularly evident. Laura Joy writes one narrative contrasting her two birth experiences, one in the hospital and one at home. Like Jennifer, she wanted a home birth after her hospital experience, seeing home birth as the counterweight to problems associated with that first birth. She explains, for example, the difference between her natural tear in an unassisted homebirth and a previous episiotomy at the hospital: "I did, unfortunately, tear, but it was much less traumatic than the huge mediolateral episiotomy that I had been given with Alyssa's birth. . . . I still often feel twinges of pain from my episiotomy scar [years later], but not from my natural tear" (Laura Joy). Laura Joy constructs the home birth as allowing her greater agency than the hospital birth (a common construction, particularly among those narratives that describe both experiences). She writes of preferring the natural home-birth tear to the carving of her body via episiotomy in the hospital. Elizabeth Grosz explains that "civilization carves meaning onto and out of bodies"; for Laura Joy, this literal carving serves as a significant reminder of the diminished agency she associates with her hospital experience. She describes her tear in the active voice ("I did . . . tear") but the cut in the passive voice (it "had been given" to her). She describes what happened in the hospital in terms of what was done to and for her, rather than of what she did, while for the home birth she describes what she did and what she chose. Her rhetorical stance grows out of these multiple experiences; her writing reflects her agency.

For Beth, whose three births have already been referenced in this chapter and in chapter 3, the solution to a traumatic first hospital birth was not to leave the hospital environment but to write a birth plan for subsequent births. For her, this creation of a rhetorical stance against one birth and in anticipation of others worked well. Beth wrote herself into a rhetorical stance—in both her birth plan and her narratives—that enabled her to come to terms with her first traumatic birth experience and write joyfully of her later births.

Rhetorical stances reveal the ways in which women mediate and remediate their birth experiences and (re)gain rhetorical agency over their births. While some women seem immediately to form a stance of acceptance, others develop a stance of resistance. Many women, despite expressing certain misgivings about technological interventions in their hospital birth stories, come to accept them by the end of their narratives; this accepting stance is evidenced by the content of the story and may be marked by use of the passive voice. These women seem to use their writing in part to come to terms with their hospital experience. This may be an example of what Robbie Davis-Floyd describes as the comforts of ritual—that is, those who "come from within a belief system" can be comforted by its rituals (190). If women read the technological interventions in hospitals as rituals of American medicine's belief system, that might explain why some women want them and how even for those who do not, these interventions can be remembered or remediated as affirming rather than intrusive.

AUTHORING MEMORY, AUTHOR AUTHORITY

> Retrospective narrativization can readily be shown to distort actual happenings.
>
> —Arthur Klineman, *The Illness Narratives*

Birth narratives derive from women's memories of their birth experiences. Experiences themselves, of course, "cannot be reproduced in speech or writing, but must instead be narrated" (Brodkey, *Academic* 83). While everyday writers generally believe their memories to be accurate, seeing their own lived experience as unassailable, narrative theorists suggest that narrating memory serves to create experiences, rather than the other way around. Remembered tales are constructed according to narrative convention (Neisser). While we may find it counterintuitive "to suggest that our anecdotes do not so much reconstitute as constitute experiences" (Brodkey, *Writing* 150), this is precisely what "the latest developments in brain science today confirm. [Which is to say that] memory, the would-be anchor of selves and lives, *constructs* the materials from the past that an earlier, more innocent view would have us believe it merely *stored*" (Eakin 106; my emphasis). To a certain extent, then, through writing a narrative about their birth experiences, women are not merely recreating those experiences but creating them. This creation is productive, with sometimes profound emotional and material results.

In viewing the creation of narrative as cathartic for the writer, we see how the body and mind work together to integrate experience and memory. Many of the women surveyed describe their reasons for writing in terms of memory; they explicitly write as a method of remembering, seeing the narrative as the "true" version:

> Writing it out helps me remember what really happened instead of a closed over version years later. (Julia, survey)
>
> I have always enjoyed writing as an "outlet" to express my feelings or "capture" a moment in time. My labor/delivery experience was so amazing & magical that I wanted to remember all the details exactally as they happened. (Amy, survey)
>
> To reflect on and so I would remember the experience better. (Marie, survey)
>
> It was cathartic for the ones that were scary experiences—a memory enhancer for those that were wonderful. (Mary, survey)

Julia writes her narrative specifically to guard against what she expects to be a "closed over version" in the future; her expectation is that the narrative written soon after the event is less subject to unwitting revision. Amy's response also reflects this belief, as she wants "to remember all the details exactally as they happened." These women believe that writing their stories will protect their memories and encapsulate the details of their experiences in a manner their brains or voices alone would not. The narratives preserve, if not *the* truth of their childbirth experience, then *a* truth, a version of memory that functions for them as received truth. Psychologists Michael Ross and Roger Buehler argue that "individuals may fill in gaps in their memories using their beliefs as guides" (207). For Ross and Buehler, memories are real but incomplete. Under this view, narratives or memories are true but fleshed out with details that match preconceived notions. As we have seen above, women write narratives that reflect their expectations, shaped by the belief systems through which they learn about and experience childbirth.

CONSTRUCTED MEMORY: MEDICAL CHARTS AS NARRATIVES

This argument would hold no more or less true for the narratives—written childbirth memories—than for medical charts, another, albeit more sanctioned, form of written childbirth memories. Obstetric charts serve myriad functions, not least as records for billing, and they reduce the rich, multilayered moments of labor and birth into precisely labeled bodily happenings and medical responses. The charts, written after the fact by medical staff, distill the experience through detached rhetorical choices—precise medical terms, abbreviations, and the agentless descriptions so common in the sciences. (For more on science and medicine's rhetorical, or arhetorical choices, see Segal, *Health* 24; and Kopelson.)

In an obstetric chart, birth choices can appear not as choices but simply as what was done, and physicians are no less likely to fill in memory gaps with beliefs than are women writing birth narratives. Medical charts are written retrospectively by individuals and so, like childbirth narratives, can be incomplete, even inaccurate, sometimes to the point that they serve as revisionist histories or justifications. My point here is not to deplore obstetric charts but to illustrate the ways in which this seemingly impersonal, factual genre parallels that of the personal birth narrative in its construction of memory and experience.

Some women's narratives tell the same basic story as the charts, although through different eyes and with different details. Other narratives, however, offer an entirely different version of events—rather than, for example, a dry, seemingly straightforward casual note stating "Pt. experienced failure to progress, c-sec indicated," a woman might describe what happened in terms of her feelings of failure or her belief that she had no choice but to have a C-section despite her wanting to give the labor more time. One narrative in particular, Jenny's, on *TheLaborofLove.com*, demonstrates the many valences a narrative can provide. Although Jenny's narrative is anomalous in many respects—in its extended length, its mixture of the present and past tense, and the postpartum research it includes—it also illustrates common features of the online birth narratives in this study. Jenny's story exhibits extremes of physical and emotional trauma in part because she experienced an undesired (and in her view, unwarranted) C-section and severe postpartum depression. I examine Jenny's narrative both to culminate this chapter and to illustrate how it reveals significant issues of memory, authority, and authorship in online birth narratives—and in any written version of events.

PRESENT TENSE/TENSION PAST: REMEMBERING IN JENNY'S STORY

Through its blend of past tense narration interspersed with feelings and thoughts in the present tense, Jenny's narrative works to preserve immediacy despite temporal and intellectual distance. She upends expectations for a straightforward story with quick shifts from past tense to present tense and to present perfect. She writes: "I asked for my room . . . Laure and Robin are both here on call! How great! . . . I was in such a fog. . . . However I'm feeling more and more nutty. . . . We turn down routine strip, IV etc and keep walking." As we see in this selection, Jenny chooses to present much of her story in the present tense. This decision reveals the mimetic nature of writing the narrative—she writes to relive the experience as much as to reconstruct what happened, and she relies on far more than her own memory to accomplish this. She completed her narrative a year after her birth experience, after conducting her own childbirth research, including extensive reading, interviewing her attendants, and reviewing her medical charts.

Jenny's story, then, is filtered through the lenses of time and others' ideas, but her writing in the present tense serves almost to mask these filters.

> It's been four hours since transition. Why don't I feel like pushing? Robin wonders. I am not even thinking about pushing, I'm just existing, waiting for this torture to end, one contraction at a time. I learn later Colleen is in the hall asking Robin CNM [certified nurse midwife] why doesn't she do something for me? I need something. Robin says I don't

> want any interference so she's not interfering. C is irritated and says she needs something. I do, I need guidance, I need to walk around and get the baby's head on the cervix. but dh[6] and I don't know that. So we just hang out on the birthing bed.

Here we see how Jenny interjects her postpartum research—about walking to try to shift the baby's placement—into the narrative. Despite writing in the present tense and thereby preserving a sense of immediacy, Jenny also offers omniscience. As an author, here, she intertwines her authority after the fact with her lack of authority during the experience; her writing serves to connect innocence and knowledge. She constructs a complex persona at once helpless and helpful, accepting and critical.

Part of Jenny's complex persona comes from her self-reflexive style. She interrupts herself in the telling of her story, drawing attention to herself as a writer: "Gee, when am I going back into past tense? Present tense is helpful some of the time." She says present tense is helpful, but in what sense? For her to remember? To relive the experience? To remediate it for her audience? Jenny provides her readers with this kind of metanarrative detail throughout her story, self-consciously reflecting on her role as an author of the narrative, of the experience. Such interjections serve to remind readers that this is a constructed story, not an experience, but also that Jenny as the author is presenting her memories to her audience thoughtfully and carefully.

When she begins to use evidence from others' writing about her birth experience, Jenny uses her authority as the author of the narrative to question authority. She both relies upon and questions the writing and memories of her birth attendants:

> [Jenny quotes here from her physician's surgical report and adds her own bracketed commentary:] "She went into active labor, progressed to full dilatation and pushed for app. four hours with crowning but definitely just caput. Sharp ischial spines[7] were noted and because of the pushing effect [?? gee folks what IS a "pushing effect"?] Pitocin was augmented to see if allowing contractions to be more powerful so that she could deliver the baby spontaneously; however, was unable to do so. She will be planned for Cesarean section." That is a direct quote.
>
> . . .
>
> You probably noted Dr. S. said "sharp ischial spines were noted." Were you wondering who noted them? So was I because they've never ever

> been noted anywhere else including not in my records from the CNMS offices. I know my spines aren't sharp. I am normal and Dr. S. just made it up because he had to put something on the report. He could care less that his words affect my entire future.
>
> . . .
>
> In 1996 when I talked with Robin she said I definitely had CPD [Cephalopelvic Disproportion] and that the DR. said the baby was never coming out right after the surgery. Interesting that she didn't remember all of that two days after birth, but could one year later. . . . When I went to talk to Wanda, the director who I thought was such a truthful and wonderful person, she told me the surgeon just forgot to put fetal distress on the surgical report when I asked her why that wasn't on there because we thought that was the reason for the surgery. . . .
>
> Another intersting detail—my baby was at +4. It's in the records. Of course I didn't realize how close he was to being born.

By placing their writing at the time against their oral descriptions at various points, Jenny challenges various authorities' memories of her childbirth story. She demonstrates the constructed nature of memories and of writing in noting the lack of stability in memories over time. The slippages, for her, denote not the fuzziness that one might expect of memories with the passage of months but fuzziness of memories after mere moments. To her this suggests disingenuousness ("Dr. S. just made it up"). When the chart supports her views, however, she does accept its veracity, as when she uses the +4 detail to disprove the CPD diagnosis. She sees memory gaps filled in with beliefs rather than with facts and uses this information to support her claim that the chart does not reflect the truth. Jenny's narrative consciously reveals potential gaps in charts.

For physicians charting after a series of medical procedures, the process of narrating any given event may begin with remembering the results and working backward to describe the causes or indications that led to those procedures or medical decisions. This may occur not because of any ill intent but simply because of time constraints or large patient loads and because doctors arrive on scene only when they are "needed"; as we see above, no physicians were with Jenny for much of her labor, so their records would necessarily cover a different time span than her own record. Charting may occur in reverse syllogistic structure: "if C-section (result), then _____ (cause)." For

Jenny, charting serves to retroactively invent reasons for procedures, and while certainly this is not always the case, she works to carefully support this claim in her own specific case. Jenny's narrative is a fitting culmination to this discussion of birth narratives in that this single story illustrates not only conflicting authority over the experience and written memories of it but also catharsis, political conviction, consumer expectations, and the formation of a stable rhetorical stance. In short, Jenny's narrative has it all.

In writing birth stories, women write themselves into the role of mother in ways that may differ from the ways they actually experienced the moments in which they became mothers—moments in which they may have been, like Jenny, (variously) positioned as agents, patients, or subjects. Online birth stories—part memoir, part political tract, part consumer testimonial—do far more than share experiences or anchor memories, and yet the sharing and documenting of their experiences is inarguably a driving impulse for these women. The urge to narrate, to (re)write one's own story, and to rely on personal experience to support, shape, and challenge others' personal decisions and opinions is not, of course, limited to women who post online birth stories. The epilogue examines the role of personal experience—and the narration of it—in academic inquiry. I argue that although academic authority does not rest in or require bodily experience, bodily experiences can nevertheless be narrated within and enhance academic work. In that spirit, the epilogue shares with readers the stories of my own childbirth experiences.

EPiLOGUE

Experiencing Birth

This book is very much wrapped up in the idea of personal experience. The personal is, of course, one way of viewing the everyday—both in terms of everyday rhetorics and everyday women, both of which are central to this book. Also, this book illustrates how experience is a complex entity with significant but never quite stable meanings for different people and audiences, as we see in chapter 5, in particular, through women's stories of and comments about their childbirth experiences. Experience and its many iterations matter in terms of how we understand feminist rhetorical agency, how we understand authority or interpret a rhetor's ethos, and how we understand the value of everyday rhetorics of health and medicine.

Part of the contribution of this book is to demonstrate the value of widening the lens of rhetorical investigations of health and medicine beyond the discourse of physicians or of interactions between patients and physicians. Using the tools of rhetorical analysis to examine a wider, messier circle of both influence on and output by individuals and across technologies is not only possible but critical for deep understanding. Also, crucially, the book encourages recognition of how women's rhetorical agency in and surrounding childbirth is sanctioned—and not sanctioned—by institutional and systemic structures and discourses beyond individual control. This exploration demonstrates that both within and despite these confines, everyday women find ways to fashion forms of rhetorical agency vis-à-vis childbirth. Women's assertions of feminist rhetorical agency do not always equate with power, however, as we see throughout this study.

This book reveals how and why contemporary women in the United States continue to take opportunities to assert feminist rhetorical agency, even if such attempts have been thwarted for others or for themselves in the past and even if that assertion is an attempt to rewrite or rewire understandings of past events. It suggests that feminist rhetorical agency can be understood as a series of disparate, collective assertions over time and space (including on the Internet and in hospitals, birthing centers, and homes), potentially effective for future women even when those individual assertions do not end with success for individual rhetors. Further, this study opens up space for explorations of the birthing rhetorics and feminist rhetorical agency asserted or achieved by women in other nations, cultures, and times, as well as by different permutations of "everyday women" in the United States.

This study has been necessarily limited, as all studies are, by the author's (which is to say, my own) capabilities, knowledges, and experiences. I share autoethnographies of my birth experiences to end this epilogue as a way of acknowledging and sharing my positionality, and yet this study rests not on the authority of my experiences but on the authority of academic inquiry. This epilogue offers readers a deep sense of my orientation to the ways experience and authority are related, and sometimes conflated, for academics as well as for birthing women and birth attendants.

EXPERIENCE, ETHOS, AND AUDIENCE-GRANTED AUTHORITY

A delightful effect of researching something as visceral and commonplace as childbirth is that when women—and men, too—discover the subject of my research, they often share birth stories with me. In elevators, hallways, and bathrooms, on telephones and over email, women have offered me glimpses into their own complicated, sometimes traumatic, sometimes inspiring birth experiences. Men, too, share their stories with me; my dentist, for example, spoke at length about his wife's four births while I was in his chair unable to reply. I welcome these stories: they are interesting; they forge connections; they affirm for me the value in studying these everyday rhetorics of childbirth. They illustrate the abiding urge to narrate experience, whether in writing or in speech. That people share these stories with me is deeply gratifying—in most situations. There have been occasions, however, when such sharing has been presented instead as a form of counterargument.

At conferences where I presented early manifestations of the arguments appearing in this book, I received the most memorable comments from women who shared their birth stories in such a way that they seemed to suggest I could not (should not) authoritatively inquire into or make claims about childbirth because I did not (then) have personal experience with it.

That is to say, these women shared their birth stories as an objection not to any argument I was making but to my very ethos in discussing the subject as a person who had not experienced childbirth. They seemed to assume my inexperience without evidence, though it was sometimes clarified with the almost-rhetorical question (or, rather, statement plus tag question), "You haven't had a baby, have you?" My examination of birth plans, in particular, was subject to criticism by women who indicated that their (bodily) experience demonstrated the futility or dangers of trying to control birth. My analysis of birth plans (early precursors to what appear here as chapters 2 and 3) was (mis)interpreted as an endorsement of them.

I now read these comments in two ways. First, I suspect my writing at those early stages was perhaps more reactionary than rhetorical: my ethos as a scholar was still developing. Second, however, I believe some mothers in my audience felt my lack of experience with childbirth made my inquiry into the subject suspicious, an ethical violation. My voice, then that of "inexperienced" woman, could not match their own—and my responses to the comments, which tended to begin and end with a perplexed but polite "Thank you for sharing your story" could not rise to the level of academic debate. I am not the only scholar to have experienced such feedback in connection to this topic, whether explicitly or more subtly. (A well-known scholar I won't name here told me she felt "persecuted" after pursuing childbirth-related research as a non-mother. A project she had originally intended as a book ended with a single article. It is in part because of her story that I write about this experience-authority issue here.)

The idea that personal/bodily experience with a topic should bolster one's claims, or even legitimize an inquiry in the first place, seems at once perfectly reasonable and perfectly absurd. (On the topic of race, for example, scholarship by members outside a studied race can be judged harshly for precisely that lack of experience, and yet scholars have and continue to do work that many find valuable on issues of race they themselves have not experienced.) On the reasonable end of the spectrum, with regard to childbirth, are many of the scholars whose work appears in this book, scholars who explicitly come to the topic of childbirth after their personal birth experiences. Suzanne Arms includes her own negative birth story in her scholarly work, as do Naomi Wolf and Robbie Davis-Floyd; Davis-Floyd also writes of a later, more empowering birth (Davis-Floyd and Dumit). Judith Leavitt says she is drawn to childbirth as an object of study because it aligns with historical changes in American health care but admits that her own pregnancy and childbirth experiences also drew her to the topic. Experience sparked Tess Cosslett's research and Della Pollock's project, too. In Pollock's case, however, the experience that began her inquiry was not precisely childbirth but hearing her first "horror story" from a stranger when she was herself visibly pregnant. Male scholars, too, can share personal tales, as Joseph Dumit does, writing with his wife about his/her/their experience with her ectopic pregnancy. For others, such as William Ray Arney and Richard Wertz, no personal experience is narrated in the text: readers do not know whether their research was instigated or affected by personal experiences with childbirth, and yet readers seem to accept their scholarship without that experience or experiential positioning.

The value of experience—and of a scholar's acknowledging or narrating that experience—depends on the audience. Ultimately, it is the audience who determines if a rhetor's ethos is appropriate, a determination that depends in part upon rhetorical conventions of particular scholarly forums and fields. And authors' worries about audiences' perceptions can prevent or color such acknowledgment. In her article about miscarriage, historian Leslie Reagan writes of how unusual it felt to share an autobiographical story at a conference. The other examples of personal stories described above include no such notion of impropriety or unease, however.

Autoethnography blurs the line between scholarly analysis and personal sharing and allows for nuances of understanding even as it may confound scholarly expectations. (Elizabeth Birmingham illustrates this hauntingly in "Another Fine Mess.") My academic, nonpersonal conference presentations early in my research on this topic were sometimes met with emotional, personal, nonacademic responses—responses that surprised and intrigued me. Some women in the conference audience seemed to expect, even to demand, personal, bodily experience as a warrant for my academic claims. I suspect those responses had to do with childbearing being so politically and ideologically charged; sometimes, when women hear another woman's story, or even scholarship about women's stories, they respond not so much to the stories or the experiences themselves so much as to the assumption that the other woman's choices and stances imply and/or require judgment of their own choices and stances.

Below I explore the interplay between two positions: experience as a legitimate, even requisite, basis for inquiry or authority, and experience as a construct, a rhetorical space that can serve to close off rather than open up discussion. My intent is not to argue for one or the other position—in fact, I consciously hover between the two. Such intentional use of ambiguity serves, I hope, to "create a space for discourse that did not exist before" so that the "ambiguity delivers an invitation to audience members to participate in the newly created discourse" (Meyer 11). I argue that scholars need not have personal experience to have the authority to inquire into topics, even bodily and contemporary topics, in part because experience itself is always something of a construct, but also because scholarly authority ultimately rests in scholarly training. At the same time, personal experience has value for scholars, and there is a potential value for readers of scholars disclosing and examining that experience when it inspires, affects, or is affected by one's scholarly work. Though I will, following the work of historian Joan W. Scott, complicate the notion of the evidence of experience, I also acknowledge experience as both inspiration and information in scholarly work.

These two positions seem contradictory, and perhaps they are, but they expose the complexity of "experience" for scholars without refuting the value of shared experience. Within English studies and outside the topic of childbirth, examples of personal experiences instigating and infusing research topics abound. Ellen Barton and Michael Bérubé, for example, both write about topics connected to issues they and their children face. Even as I question the stability of experience, I affirm that acknowledging one's positioning can be of value to readers as they evaluate arguments (see Sullivan and Porter 75; Kirsch). To put this belief into practice, I conclude with autoethnographic narratives of my own two birth experiences, refracting them through the arguments made and discoveries shared in previous chapters. I examine the rhetorical and material effects of my research on my birth choices, in hopes that this reflection can shed light on my own positioning and help readers to engage with my work with both a scholarly distance and an interpersonal familiarity. By writing my own birth stories in this forum, I also seek to deepen my connection to the women in this study, whose stories sustained and inspired not only this project but also my own and other women's birth experiences.

EXPERIENCE: REQUIREMENT VERSUS CONSTRUCT

> Just as nature is one of culture's most startling and non-innocent products, so is experience one of the least innocent, least self-evident aspects of historical, embodied movement.
>
> —Donna Haraway, *Simians, Cyborgs, and Women*

Women in this study write extensively about experience. They write of experiences they desire(d), of not having experience, of wanting to learn from others' experiences, of basing plans for future births on the experience of their first. The idea that childbirth is an ordinary and relatively predictable event is belied by the fact that for the women in this study, the idea of a childbirth "experience" as unique to each woman (and each birth) is absolute. One woman, Sherry, writes, "After much research and discussion with my husband, Brett, we decided that we would want a childbirth experience that had minimal intervention and the best way to approach this desire would be to hire a midwife and plan for a homebirth." Sherry's emphasis on a particular "experience" is commonplace in the narratives.

For the women in this study, childbirth is an experience: an individual, nonstandard event. The desire for a particular experience is fueled by women's epistemologies and situations but also by their educational knowledge of other women's experiences gained through reading or conversation. Such knowledge is acquired in part through online birth narratives—as survey responses like Cynthia's attest: "While I was planning my birth choices, I wanted to read about other [women's birth] experiences." Women I surveyed relied upon narratives to learn about birth and later posted their narratives online so they could share stories of their bodily experiences with others. They hoped their (bodily) experiences could provide others with (educational) experience: "I wanted to share my story so that other mothers-to-be could read and learn from my experience" (Jessica, survey); "I wanted to share my 'bizarre' experience" (Mary, survey).

For their first births, as we see in chapter 2, women make plans based in large part on reading and research—their educational knowledge; for subsequent births, however, they explicitly rely on their bodily experience(s) giving birth. For births beyond the first, comments like these are common: "The second time around, my expectations were mainly based on my first experience" (Anna, survey); "I had such a good experience with induction the first time, we decided to be induced" (Julie). Childbirth is imagined, researched, planned, monitored, and recorded, but a woman's own bodily experience of childbirth seems to trump any other form of knowledge or experience. Upon acquiring this bodily experience, women feel they have gained authority and want to share the stories of their experiences. (And this may explain those conference reactions I got from women who, when provided with what seemed like a public opportunity to share their own birth stories, took it.)

As I demonstrate in chapter 5, writing a birth story can accomplish multiple goals at once, goals prioritized in different ways by different women. Women write for themselves, achieving catharsis, but they also write for others in an effort to inform, guide, and connect with other women. They write their birth stories not solely to "remember" their birth experiences but also, to a certain extent, to *create* those memories and thereby in a sense to retroactively create those experiences. Birth narratives mediate women's expectations for and experiences with birth. Nowhere in this cycle of experience sought, remembered, and shared, however, is an explicit recognition of experience as a construct of memory. "Construct," here, means built with memory and ideology, for memory's lacunae are bridged by beliefs (Ross and Buehler 207). For the women in this study—and, notably, for those women who invoked their experience at conferences—bodily experience, or at least their narrated memory of that experience, serves as an unassailable form of evidence.

Many women—in birth stories, online birth missives, and casual conversations—sometimes jokingly, sometimes seriously suggest that perhaps male physicians shouldn't deliver babies because they don't (can't) have the bodily experience of childbirth themselves and couldn't possibly understand what it's like. Such comments would indicate that the bodily experience of childbirth should be a prerequisite for attending birth, that bodily experience trumps, or at least crucially complements, educational knowledge—as my conference combatants would perhaps agree. Such comments focus on male physicians who *cannot* experience childbirth. Meanwhile, female physicians, while potentially capable of giving birth, are certainly not required to have experienced it to attend births. (And given the demands and expectations of medical students, residents, and interns, many do not have children until their careers are well established.) Midwives, on the other hand, were historically required to have given birth—to have had the bodily experience of childbirth—as a prerequisite to training (Borst). Further, midwives traditionally trained through apprenticeship, participating in women's deliveries for years before attending one as a midwife. As William Ray Arney puts it, "Experience was the teacher of most midwives" (22), "experience" here referring to midwives' experience attending births. It is worth noting that attending a birth provides a different kind of bodily knowledge than giving birth does and a different kind of knowledge than educational knowledge gained through reading does.

Although having given birth is not a requirement today, many midwives still do come to the profession after having children. Bodily experience with birth, then, may offer one way of distinguishing among different types of childbirth attendants. Judy Barrett Litoff marks the nurse-midwife as a more medical (educational) than experiential practitioner, the basis for her authority somewhat like a physician's in that sense. The prototypical nurse-midwife, with a reliance upon educational knowledge but with skills and an orientation more woman-centered than a physician's, occupies a kind of third space between the prototypical roles/poles along the spectrum between lay midwife and obstetrician in terms of conceptual and rhetorical alignment with valuing bodily or educational knowledge. (See Taylor for more detail on the complex role of nurse-midwives in various birthing contexts.) And yet while there are expected roles for each of these types of birth attendants, any individual birth attendant may draw on different types of knowledge and experience in different situations—and with different birthing mothers or in different rhetorical spaces.

Lay midwife Mary Welcome tells investigative journalist Jessica Mitford that experience as a birth attendant, along with a modicum of educational knowledge, prepares a midwife and grants her authority: "'I think that after you've done a hundred deliveries, if you have a little bit of theory along with it, that would be sufficient. The main thing about birth is the experience of knowing what to do in difficult situations and anticipating what might go wrong. Experience is the whole thing'" (qtd. in Mitford 196). Welcome's idea of experience is clearly that of bodily experience as an attendant—experience as an observer and helper rather than bodily experience giving birth. Perhaps ironically, her definition would suggest that physicians (of either sex) could also be prepared through experiences attending births. (Recall, however, that physicians do not typically train by attending births as observers or helpers for years the way lay midwives do. Physicians' birth attendance is temporally limited in ways midwives' attendance is typically not. Responsible for many patients at once, physicians often visit laboring women only for the delivery itself and for sporadic exams at the later stages of labor rather than stay with women throughout their labors.)

"Experience" seems to signify in multiple and competing ways. As chapter 3 reveals, women bring different kinds of knowledge—bodily, experiential, educational—to their birth preparation. But each of those categories of knowledge could be simultaneously expanded and split to include bodily experience as an attendant versus bodily experience as a birthing woman, educational experience as an observer versus educational experience gained through reading, lecture, and memorization. Experience is at the heart of women's choices in birth attendants—and by this I mean not only women's perceptions of the attendant's experience but also the experience the woman has with the attendant.

The value of experience is significant for both birthing women and childbirth practitioners but must not be confused with the value of experience for scholarly inquiry about childbirth. The work of physicians and midwives in childbirth—physically present and responsible attendants at a life-altering event—can hardly be compared to the work of scholars, work produced on computers in coffee shops, offices, and libraries, far from the bloody, heady moments of childbirth itself. And yet, when scholars are confronted about their bodily experiences rather than (or even in addition to) their intellectual arguments, there seems to be an expectation that bodily experience should authorize scholarly inquiry into certain topics. Arguments about a birth attendant's bodily experience with childbirth, or lack thereof (or educational knowledge, or lack thereof), resonate more than arguments about a scholar's experiential qualifications for an inquiry into childbirth discourse. The tacit knowledge one may gain and draw upon through bodily experience matters significantly more for a full-body experience such as childbirth than for the always already partial renderings any scholar can provide through words alone.

One of the most significant reasons, however, that experience must not be considered a prerequisite for scholarly work is that experience is itself so amorphous a concept. Another's experience is impossible to truly understand for the very reason it is invoked: because it belongs to someone else. As Shannon, a woman I surveyed, puts it: "I knew I couldn't compare or base my experience off what happened to someone else . . . simply because they weren't me and I wasn't them." But even one's own experience—or, perhaps more accurately, one's own memory of experience—is necessarily incomplete, shifting depending on context, changing over time. As Linda Brodkey suggests in *Academic Writing as Social Practice*, experience can be shared *only* through narration. And narration relies on memory, which is itself at a further remove from experience.

Although this story telling can serve multiple purposes, the stories of experience will always be, in Donna Haraway's words, "an intentional construction" (*Simians* 113). As chapter 5 illustrates, a birth story is multivalenced, accomplishing multiple goals simultaneously. It is also always a construction, as Jenny's story—the extended story that concludes that chapter—vividly illustrates. Experience in narrative form is built with a combination of memory and belief, based on reflection and set in relief (in the architectural sense of standing out).

Because this construction is always also partial and contingent upon circumstances and subject positions, relying upon personal experience as a position from which to evaluate scholarship is a problematic stance. (We know, for example, that while scholars have done important and well-received research into sensitive race issues, a scholar's race and ethnicity can provide or complicate both entrée and reception. See Heath; Prendergast, "Race.") Experience and scholarship can connect and inform one another, as they do in autoethnographies and any scholarly work that acknowledges experiential underpinnings; the two can, perhaps, converse, but one cannot easily be invoked to evaluate the other. Arguments from stories of personal experience can engage only with particular aspects of scholarly inquiry, just as the story a scholar tells through his or her research can engage only with particular aspects of experience. The conversation a scholar begins or continues with his or her work can include stories of experience, but personal experience alone, while valuable as an educational tool, is an incomplete contribution to a scholarly conversation.

I have come to see (my) experiences with childbirth as a way of concluding, of describing how different knowledges (for me) converge in the delivery room (in my case, my living room in Illinois for one birth, my bathtub in Rhode Island for another) and affected my own sense of agency. Inscribing my own birth experiences serves as a way of reflecting on what I've written in and learned from writing this book and as a way of responding, post facto, to those women who challenged my earlier lack of experience. I am pleased that I gave birth and believe these stories enhance my work here, but I remain adamant that I did not need to give birth to legitimize this research project. I did not, after all, have a baby in service of my scholarship. The decision was personal, not professional. And yet I feel compelled to share the story of the experiences here.

My own experiences were shaped by my absorption of other women's narrated experiences and reflections. My research and writing on this topic delimited and circumscribed my choices—or, rather, significantly expanded my options and deepened my sense of options beyond those usually ascribed to birthing women in our society. I have broken the autoethnographic portion of this chapter into three parts, each with a subtitle inspired by and intended to echo the types of titles of the online birth stories in my study.

MY FIRST PREGNANCY: DEFYING EXPECTATIONS

During the years I spent researching and writing this book, I conceived, carried, and gave birth to two children. As my pregnancy and childbirth years overlapped my research and writing process, the life experiences and research/writing experiences inevitably affected each other. The story I offer is autobiographical, but it is more than that: "Autoethnography is an autobiographical genre of writing and research that displays multiple levels of consciousness, connecting the personal to the cultural" (Ellis and Bochner 739). In this case, I connect the personal not only to the cultural but also to the textual, making direct reference to the research and analysis presented throughout this book. I reflect on the ways this project shaped my own assertions of feminist rhetorical agency over my births.

For both births I chose home birth. I did not do so out of a wholesale rejection of the medical progress narrative (see chapter 1) but because of my sincere belief, particularly after conducting the birth plan research for this project and reading hundreds of online birth stories, that the birth I wanted was most readily achievable at home, away from hospital hierarchies and control. For women in this study who birthed at home, unpleasant hospital experiences often drove later choices to birth at home. Representative is this sentiment from the survey: "I hated the whole hospital experience. When we got pregnant again, I at first thought I would use a lay midwife for labor support for another hospital birth. Soon we decided we could do it ourselves at home safely" (Daryl). I wanted to labor where I felt comfortable, knowing that for me my very entry into a hospital would bring along unnecessary stress and fear—and therefore pain.

I also wanted to labor and deliver in the same safe place without having to deal with traffic, waiting rooms, or insurance forms. I wanted to know my labor attendants, and I wanted them with me for my entire labor. I wanted my labor to progress at its own pace, minimally affected by the clock or protocols. While I wanted assistance with pain, I wanted it in the form of continuous social support rather than numbing medications. And most of all, I wanted my baby to be born in my home, with its yellow walls, soft lighting, and plentiful plants. In short, I wanted many options that a hospital birth simply could not provide and other options that hospital births tend not to provide. I also, of course, wanted a safe birth, with medical assistance available if necessary. For me, these desires were met by the proximity of hospital(s) to my home, the ready availability of 911 emergency service, and my trust in my midwife to know if or when assistance beyond her expertise was warranted.

I chose a lay midwife, a certified professional midwife. I did so despite the fact that the nearest practicing CPM I could find was three hours away in another state, which was less than convenient for prenatal visits and less than reassuring in terms of concerns about a quick labor. (This latter point was felt particularly poignantly by my husband, Luke, who, although incredibly supportive of my desire to home birth, was understandably wary of potentially having to deal with my labor and birth alone while our midwife sped along the highway.) Home birth was also not covered by our insurance.

For most women in the United States, home birth is not a viable option, in part because of cost. Because most insurance companies do not cover it, individuals who choose home birth often pay more out-of-pocket than those who choose hospital births, despite the true cost of home birth being significantly cheaper than the true cost of even nonsurgical hospital births. Also, home birth is rarely seriously considered because of the misinformation that circulates around its dangers. Home birth is, in short, associated with a dangerous past (one that is—in part, at least—a received fiction, as I demonstrate in chapter 2), a past that hospital birth is viewed as having alleviated. As a landmark study performed in the United States and published in the *British Medical Journal* finds, however, planned home birth with CPMs is at least as safe as hospital birth, with far fewer interventions (Johnson and Daviss). Worth noting is that the documentary *The Business of Being Born* has contributed to a slight uptick in home births and to a shift in the national conversation about home birth (see Hensley Owens, "Reviews and Reactions").

Many of my family members did not greet my choice of birth attendants enthusiastically. By the sixth week of my pregnancy, I seemed to have become "the vessel" that early modern texts talk of: some of my closest and dearest relatives referred to my choice as "endangering their niece/nephew/grandchild [insert appropriate future kinship title here]." For those who most vociferously objected, there was no interest in my wishes, my reasons, or my knowledge(s). Unquestioning acceptance of the medical model of childbirth and the progress narrative of science and medicine ruled their reactions. I was even accused, at the end of my first trimester, of irresponsibly "not receiving prenatal care" because I had not yet seen an obstetrician and, most egregiously, to their minds, had not had an ultrasound. To my mind, however, my prenatal care had already been extensive: beyond visiting my midwife to have my blood pressure checked, uterus palpated, and stomach measured, I had also dutifully been taking prenatal vitamins, given up alcohol, adapted my exercise regimen, and adjusted my diet.

My decision early in my second trimester to have an ultrasound was greeted with relief; my report that a reading based on a machine had confirmed not only my pregnancy but the presence and proper function of baby's basic organs trumped any assurance I could offer. I had initially planned to avoid an ultrasound, partly because I did not feel it necessary, having read (too much) about their potential use for misdiagnosis (Cartwright; Goer; Dumit and Sensiper), and partly because I knew that the ultrasound administrator would likely know the sex of the baby before I did (we wanted to wait until the birth to find out). I did not like the idea of someone else having this knowledge, even if it was not shared with me.

I ultimately decided to have an ultrasound, however, because I had become obsessed with a particular fear, one caused in part by a dream and one that I could easily put to rest by seeing the digital image but otherwise would have had to live with until the moment of birth. For those curious as to the precise fear: at the end of Ina May Gaskin's *Spiritual Midwifery* is a poignant story of a baby born without a skull. Neither parents nor birth attendants knew of the problem until the birth. The baby was birthed safely but could not live. The baby was initially placed in the hospital, where nurses were instructed not to feed it because it would die anyway. The parents, objecting to that plan, soon took their child home, feeding and loving the baby until its inevitable demise. I dreamed that my baby was, like that one, perfectly healthy in utero, with one glaring and insurmountable exception: the lack of a skull.

After the dream, I simply could not be calmed until I knew with reasonable certainty that my baby had a skull. And so I fit into what Lisa Mitchell and Eugenia Georges identify (for North American women, in contrast to Greek women) as embedding ultrasound technology within an "individualized ideology of risk and maternal responsibility" (119). While my particular fear resulted from perhaps an overabundance of information—because of this project, I was far more familiar than most women with bizarre and horrific, though incredibly rare, potential problems—fear among pregnant women is hardly anomalous. Though I was also more familiar than perhaps most American women with what William Ray Arney terms the "residual normalcy" of birth (51), I was not inoculated from fears of the unknown. Unlike some women, I did not feel that the pregnancy was more "real" after the ultrasound, a phenomenon Barbara Duden has described as "technological quickening" (qtd. in Mitchell and Georges 106), but I was able to move beyond my irrational fear, which was profoundly important to me.

I was also, however, disappointed with the ultrasound technician's treatment of our decision not to learn the sex. After our quick, firm, and united response of "no" to the singsong question, "Do you want to know the se-ex?" we were greeted with another singsong, this time laced with disappointment, "Okaaa-ay . . ." Alone, these phrases would be inconsequential, but they were followed after the ultrasound with, "Okay, now *I* know the sex of your baby, but I won't tell you"—and here she looked up pointedly, as if giving us one more chance to change our minds—"and I won't even write it down. I'll forget, so no one will know." This reinforcement of her knowledge exceeding ours, and her power over that knowledge's dissemination, was somewhat upsetting. I also suspected that her firm conviction about the sex meant it was a boy, since girl pronouncements are typically made rather tentatively at that early stage. This suspicion inevitably affected my expectations about the sex of my future child for the duration of my pregnancy, no matter how hard I tried to forget or dismiss the interaction. (My child is indeed a boy, though of course I can never know for sure if the technician's description would have been the same if I were carrying a girl.)

I did see an obstetrician ("Finally, a *doctor*!" certain family members would say) at regularly spaced intervals during my pregnancy, which was part of the standard of care for my midwife's practice. I consented to standard blood tests and a GBS (Group B strep) test—I say "consented" purposefully here, for as a home-birth midwifery patient, such tests were offered to me as options, whereas to the obstetrician's usual patients, they were routine, required. My pregnancy, then, was monitored in both the most "traditional," as in age-old, methods by my midwife and many of the most "traditional," as in medicalized, technologically advanced, methods known. For me, this combination honored my trust in the holistic midwifery model (Lay) and allowed me to take advantage of what I felt were relevant aspects of Western medicine without compromising my reluctance to allow the medical model of childbirth to dictate the process. This balance worked well for me, despite the inconveniences that resulted from my engaging such distant caregivers and planning a somewhat alegal birth. (In Illinois, while it is legal for women to give birth at home, it is illegal for a CPM to attend a home birth, and almost no physicians and very few CNMs will attend home births.)

Because my desires matched so perfectly with my midwife's standards of care, described in a detailed email and handout, my plans for the birth did not coalesce into a written birth plan. I reasoned that if I had to transfer to a hospital, most of my desires would be (always already) contradicted by my very presence there even if the plan *were* respected. Also, it seemed unlikely that either my written or oral wishes would be much respected given that I would have to first somehow explain my home labor, which I would have to do without mention of my illegal midwife. I expected that if a hospital transfer were required, I would have even less agency in the hospital than most birthing women.

FALSE LABOR, FAST HOME BIRTH

Enough background. After a twenty-two-hour doula-attended "false" labor, which left me dilated to four centimeters, partially effaced, and fully frustrated, I waited two weeks, through and well past my due date. Eventually my midwife (whom I'll call Elizabeth) suggested stripping my membranes to get things (re)started.[1] I agreed somewhat warily at first but cottoned to the idea as I became more and more uncomfortable being super-pregnant. (I also caught a glimpse of what some women who request C-sections must feel. Here the evidence of experience seems unassailable. Had I never been forty-one weeks pregnant myself, I don't think I could have comprehended, much less so readily empathized with, that desire.) On the appointed day, we drove the three hours to see Elizabeth, and the stripping of membranes was uncomfortable but not excruciating—a perception I attribute to my midwife's expertise and gentle touch.

Following what proved to be our last meal as non-parents (lovely Indian food—we almost-seriously considered naming a girl Makhani, after the dish *dal makhani*), Luke and I drove home and went to sleep expecting "something to happen" in the night. At 4 A.M. I woke with a full bladder, and upon standing up my water broke—not in a huge gush, as in the movies, but with the trickle my midwife had described as a possibility, so I knew what was happening. I called Elizabeth, who told me my contractions would start soon and to call her again once I'd had a few rounds of those. Maybe three minutes later I was hit with a contraction—and finally I understood why everyone had told me that when the contractions came "for real" I would *just know.* I had somehow scoffed at that, particularly after the false labor with what I had thought were hard contractions—hard enough that I'd had to stop while walking and pause while talking. But these were completely different: a creeping, yanking sensation from deep inside me I can only describe as more than physical. They left me breathless from the start, lasted about a minute, and were four minutes apart.

I called Elizabeth again, and she sent her apprentices on their way (a three-hour drive). Not ten minutes later I was back on the phone, telling Elizabeth that the contractions were now three minutes apart and that they were "kicking my ass" already. She said she was on her way. My mom, in town hoping to catch the birth, was given the task of baking chocolate chip cookies—I had planned to make them myself as a labor project, following my midwife's advice and planning to be like the Amish women she delivered, but couldn't at that point. I couldn't imagine a better comfort food for labor, though as it turned out I didn't want to eat anything—even a cookie—until after the birth.

I knew the labor was going to be fast, partly based on my mother's experience (after all, I was nearly born in a VW) but mostly because of the way the contractions felt and how close they were. I just knew, and I was worried that help wouldn't get there in time. At this point Luke woke up, hearing me talking on the phone, and I told him it was time to rock and roll—we were finally having a baby! I was so excited when I told him! (I was in between contractions, so excitement was possible. During contractions I couldn't do a thing but try to hang on to myself.) Sweet Luke, not so good on lack of sleep and assuming labor would be slow, rolled over and went back to sleep. A few minutes later, after my worst contraction up to that point, I went back and told him he really needed to get up, to help me fill the pool, and so on—he was very good about that.

At this point, the memories start getting a little fuzzy. (When faced with such fuzziness, I no doubt fill gaps in my memory with beliefs, with what I imagine happened based on what I have come to "know" about birth, as discussed in chapter 5 with regard to physicians when charting and with regard to other women when writing their birth narratives.) The contractions were hard, harder than I can describe or even remember, and I tried out the birth/labor pool in an effort to relax. I imagined sweet relief in that water, which is what countless books and online narratives suggested would await me there. What I got instead was intense, stabbing pain. (Here, not for the last time, my bodily experience shattered my educational knowledge.)

The water, which makes things move along more quickly, was no relief to me at that point (which I later realized was already the stage known as "transition"—the final two centimeters of dilation and the most painful part of labor) and was instead like a punishment. I would stay in for one or two contractions and try to take advantage of my weightlessness to move around, but then it would be too much and I'd get out again, running (well, not running, in my state—more like urgent waddling) to the bathroom, which seemed like the safest place in the world. I would sit on the toilet and feel safe, and when a contraction hit I'd stand up, lean on the counter, groan, end up on the floor—I'd say prone, but with the belly it wasn't quite that, more like a yogic child's pose—and groan some more. Luke would follow and encourage me: "You can do this, honey." I went back and forth from pool to bathroom for probably an hour and a half, and then Elizabeth's apprentices showed up. I was naked, my hair a mess, nothing like the relaxed, excited, very together version of myself they'd met at my "false" labor—we joked about that until the next contraction hit, and I went back into the pool for a few contractions, this time relying on Luke's gaze to get me through. When even that stopped working, I blew bubbles.

I looked up from the pool's edge to see one of the apprentices doing cross-stitch or something and almost despaired. No, I did despair. I figured she somehow knew we were in for a long wait, and I didn't know how I could possibly handle this longer, especially not if it was going to get harder still. But when that contraction was over, that apprentice asked if I'd like to be checked—and I answered with an enthusiastic and yet frightened "Yes!" I lay on a disposable pad draped over our brightly striped living room rug and soon she announced, and I'll never forget this, "Well, there's good news and then there's good news." Excellent! I think she actually meant good and bad, but she definitely said good and good. I was fully dilated—her words were, "Your cervix is gone"—and ready to push, but Elizabeth still wasn't there. But then all of a sudden Elizabeth appeared, and they were setting up a birth stool and covering the floor with disposable pads. My contractions had temporarily gone away—a delightful phase Sheila Kitzinger calls the "rest and be thankful" part of labor (which I mentioned, apparently feeling the need to show off my book knowledge). At this point cameras came out, Luke called our friend Janine to help, and my mom abandoned the cookie project to take up a place at my feet, where she remained to smile me through the rest of my labor—a more delighted, inspiring cheerleader could not be imagined. I started off sitting on a birth stool with Luke behind me.

I had to push for an hour and a half, and this was much harder than I'd anticipated, and not as intuitive as I'd imagined, either. I'd puff out my air as I "pushed," and they'd tell me to use the air to push, not to waste it. (See Jordan, *Birth*, on Yucatan women's mouths being covered with birth attendants' hands to keep their breath in their bodies for just this purpose—I'd read that before giving birth but didn't remember it until rereading it years after this birth experience.) There were encouraging voices all around, and they'd check the baby's heartbeat with a handheld Doppler after every push. I asked a few times if things were okay, but really I could hear the heartbeat myself and was comforted by the pulsing, liquidy sound. When they were quiet I'd ask them to encourage me—I had a voice and used it during this phase, even right during contractions, whereas before I'd have been hard pressed to say anything coherent at all. Elizabeth let me move as I wished, but it was pretty clear that she thought I should be on my back. At one point I blurted, "But the books say that won't work!" (or maybe it was "But the books say that'll hurt more!"—something like that).

She laughed back at me, "The books are wrong!"—a delightful and yet difficult thing to hear as a person studying childbirth texts and wanting to give birth "right," or at least in an appropriately emancipated, feminist, agentful manner. Here was my illegal midwife telling me it was okay to break those rules (the ones I interpreted as intended to be breaking other "rules," if that makes any sense). I also agreed to a quick catheter at some point, after discovering that I simply could not rid myself of all the water I'd been drinking. My midwife suggested that my full bladder could be impeding the pushing. The catheter was offered, not insisted upon, which I liked, and although I had thought I'd hate a catheter, it was a quick little thing—just a tiny temporary tube that gave me instant relief.

Moments after the catheter, after an extremely difficult push, one of the midwife's apprentices cheered, "You've given birth to a hair!"

"All that for a *hair*?!" I barked in frustration.

But then the head was out, and my baby was in my arms. (More time passed in between, but that's all I remember.) I asked "Is he okay?" before anyone mentioned the sex: a boy, as we'd expected. There was a call for blankets and my body was shaking—apparently so much that Janine, who'd seen two births before, told me later she was alarmed. My mom thought I was cold, but I didn't feel cold, just happy. Elizabeth explained that the shaking was the adrenaline "taking care of itself."

Birthing the placenta is a blur, and then we were alone with our baby, staring in wonder and attempting a first breast-feeding latch. The birth attendants had respectfully retreated while they inspected the placenta. When they returned moments later, they rather excitedly showed it to us. It had a slight abnormality that had Elizabeth fascinated—she has something of an obsession with placentas (I mean that quite seriously; she's working on a coffee table book with pictures of placentas). This abnormality, while not a problem for my birth, could have been somewhat disastrous had I given birth in a hospital setting, where my "false" labor could easily have been deemed an arrested one, given my dilation to four centimeters. Had they then broken my waters to "speed things along," as commonly happens (though it may not be effective; see Goer 239), the abnormality—a larger-than-usual blood vessel and an extra lobe—could have become a liability. If popped, my midwife explained, that vessel would have led to a life-threatening situation for the baby and a C-section for me. The abnormality, then, which an ultrasound wouldn't have caught and which I could never have known about, affirms my belief that for me, a home birth was the best option.[2]

MORE FALSE LABOR, EVEN FASTER SECOND HOME BIRTH

While my choices for the second birth were quite different due to location, availability of midwives, and finances (ironically, I had more financial resources available for a home birth as a graduate student in central Illinois than I did as a tenure-track professor living in New England), I again chose a home birth. This time the midwife was a nurse-midwife approved as an "out-of-network" provider by my insurance.[3] And unlike the first experience, this midwife lived ten minutes from my home, and most of my prenatal appointments were at my house.

As with my first child, my second child made her nearly-ready-to-be-born presence known regularly and intensely in the form of so-called false labors. Beginning two weeks before my estimated due date and continuing until the eventual birth over a week past it, I experienced regular, significant contractions about every other day. At three minutes apart, lasting a minute, and increasing in intensity over the course of an hour or more, I would often suspect that *this* labor was "real." (Despite all my educational knowledge and previous bodily experience with "false" labor, I still found myself regularly turning to a handout in the booklet I'd been given at an appointment early in my pregnancy, at an OB's office before I'd found a local midwife. The handout offers a chart to help women distinguish between "True Labor" and "False Labor.")

According to the handout, contractions coming in regular intervals, getting closer and stronger, signify true labor. My contractions would begin just over three minutes apart, then come closer. The handout says that in true labor, walking makes contractions stronger; in false labor, it does not. (I challenge any nine-months pregnant woman to go for a walk while experiencing strong contractions and not at least think the contractions are getting stronger.) In true labor, the handout assures, contractions are "usually felt in lower back and radiate to the front"; in false labor, contractions are "usually felt in fundus and groin." My memory of Ethan's birth suggested to me that these sensations are not universal—my true labor then had felt more like this false labor description, and vice versa. This distinction combined with my experiential, bodily knowledge confused me further. The handout notes that lying down does not make true labor go away—and of course it doesn't (but I also know that lying down *can* slow early true labor down). This last bit of distinction proved helpful many times, as I would wonder if I was in labor and try to remember the bodily sensation of my previous labor, only to recall that I never really experienced early labor, only the hard labor after my water broke. So I'd decide this "could be it," call Luke at work, drink a glass of water, lie down, and wait . . . Sometimes the contractions would continue at a regular clip for thirty minutes or an hour, my anticipation rising before disappointment (or relief) set in as the contractions would get farther apart and less intense.

Because my first labor had moved so quickly, my midwife encouraged me to call her whenever I felt contractions. She wanted to be sure she was ready in case my labor was "precipitous" (lasting fewer than two hours). But this careful acknowledgment of my probable short labor meant I was calling my midwife nearly every forty-eight hours, saying, "Well, they're three minutes apart, and more intense than last time, but I'm lying down now, so we'll see . . . I'll call you back in a half hour." Eventually I stopped calling her, feeling like the proverbial Peter, calling "Baby?!" instead of "Wolf!"

As with my first, this baby seemed determined to wait until my mother arrived. On a Friday evening we drove the half hour to Providence to pick her up, stopping first for a dinner of Indian food—chicken tikka masala, for those who will insist on attributing my next-day labor to that evening's meal. That night I slept fitfully, awakened at 3 A.M. by still more "false" contractions—although a better term might be "practice." A predawn walk around the block left me feeling something had changed, and a cleaning frenzy later that day solidified my sense that labor really was imminent this time. That morning my midwife visited for a prenatal appointment, finding us in the garden. I measured four centimeters dilated and 80 percent effaced but with no contractions at exam time: not in labor.

We all took an afternoon nap, and then Luke went to the grocery store to buy the spaghetti I had requested for dinner. My mother took my son for a walk to the park; I was to meet them on their walk back. Realizing I was alone in the house, a rare occasion since becoming a parent, I blasted the stereo and scrubbed the bathroom, swept the floors, and dusted shelves with Aretha Franklin and Gillian Welch marking time for me. At some point I began having contractions again, but I purposely ignored them, cleaning and dancing through them. Around five thirty I began the walk to the park and at this point realized the full force of that "walking makes them stronger" distinction between true and false labor. I could hardly take a step when the contractions were happening, though I walked fairly well in the intervening time. Resting on a rock, I timed the contractions. Three minutes apart, again.

I called my mother, who was rather inexplicably lost with Ethan in the five blocks between my house and the park. We eventually met up, and though I made no mention of my probable status, my mother noticed the look on my face when I slowed to a near stop during contractions. Having learned her lesson from baby #1 (or perhaps because baby #1 was present as a distraction in the form of an almost-three-year-old) she did not pester me for information; we simply made our way home. I had two heaping platefuls of spaghetti with red sauce and green beans, a favorite childhood meal, and just as I was finishing, Ethan announced, "There's a baby at the door."

A bit startled, because I still hadn't mentioned that I was fairly certain I really was in labor this time, I said to him, "I think you're right," and then casually said I was going to go call Michelle (the midwife). (I'll also mention here that Brigitte Jordan writes in *Birth in Four Cultures* that in the Yucatan, midwives commonly utter sentences like "Push, push now, the baby is at the door" when a woman is giving birth.) That phone call placed (during which the midwife said she was going to take a nap, a response that concerned me more than a little), Mom gave Ethan a bath while Luke and I timed my contractions and wondered if this was really it.

Just as Ethan got out of the tub, the contractions got cracking in a serious and completely unignorable way. I rocked on the floor on my hands and knees, begging Luke to call Michelle again and get her over to the house, STAT. Ethan saw me on the floor and cheerfully climbed onto my back. I accepted his slight body weight gratefully for one cycle of contractions, but by the next I implored my mother to take him upstairs to bed. Child kissed, mother absent, I proceeded to the bathtub. While I had not intended to labor in the tub, having not particularly enjoyed the water-immersed moments of my first birth, I nonetheless felt I simply had to be in the tub immediately. Once in the water, the contractions only got stronger, and I knew the baby was coming soon. I groaned and moaned and tried to make things feel like they had the time before. I wanted Luke's calm eyes to guide me, and they were there—helpful, though somehow not quite as helpful as the first time. I remembered my mantra—"I feel calm. I can do this. And then I get to have a baby!"—which soothed me, but then I forgot it. I worried that Michelle wouldn't make it. I worried I couldn't do it this time. And I didn't WANT to do it. I remember thinking, "Why is birth so hard?"

When Michelle arrived, I hardly noticed—there was a blood pressure check, I think, things like that, but I remained in the tub. She was on hand to remind me to make low-pitched noises rather than the whiny squeals that slid up the scale in a few near-panicky moments. Her presence was calming and unobtrusive; only later did I learn that she and her assistant had arrived with a whole mess of just-in-case equipment I never even saw.

At one point I left the bathtub, determined to get away from the pain, to simply leave it behind. I kept asking where I could go, and both midwife and assistant sweetly offered different places in the house. It was Luke who figured out what I meant and reminded me that I couldn't get away from it. So I got back in the tub.

I still didn't intend to give birth in my bathtub in what I joke is the smallest bathroom in the world (it is), and yet moments later that's exactly what I was doing. It felt interminable, the pushing stage, but in reality it lasted no more than twenty minutes. I repeatedly asked when it would be over, and Michelle encouraged, "Soon." Once the baby's head was out, her body slipped gracefully into Michelle's arms and then immediately into mine. I nursed the pink-blue darling for a few minutes as my blood pressure was checked and my uterus palpated, not realizing we didn't know the sex until my mother asked excitedly from the doorway, "Well, what do we have?!" I think Luke announced it was a girl, and we both cried with the surprise of that (all the "old wives' methods" had suggested "boy") and with relief that the hard part was over. I still had to birth the placenta, which I think I did while standing in the tub, and then I was helped to the office/guest room. (No one told me one isn't to climb stairs for several days after giving birth, so my upstairs bedroom but downstairs bathroom became a bit of an issue; happily, my mom didn't mind our taking over "her" guest bed and sleeping in our room.)

While I continued to nurse or watch a sleeping baby rest on my chest (baby measurements and the like waited at least an hour), Michelle noted that her inspection of the placenta revealed a missing piece. She was concerned that the piece remained within me, which would be a dangerous complication. I worried over this, submitted to rather painful uterine palpations, and tried to determine how much bleeding was normal versus "too much," but before long she found the missing piece in the bathtub, and all was well. When I went to the bathroom, I started to clean up a bit of blood and was stopped by the midwife and her assistant, who insisted they would clean up. I have never been so grateful in my life, and my tub has never been so clean. I returned to the futon to find a shirtless Luke holding a newly clean baby. They weighed her (8 lb., 2 oz.), measured her, and filled out paperwork (including a delightful mistake—Michelle noted that I had gained twenty-five pounds in pregnancy, which is quite a bit less than I actually gained, but I didn't correct her, amused by the happy number). They went over postpartum instructions and tucked the three of us into bed. Michelle said she'd be by in the morning to check on us, and then she was gone. Luke and I drifted off to sleep with Eleni Lucía between us for the first of many shared nights.

REFLECTIONS

Even as I write what I believe to be the truest version of my experiences giving birth, I acknowledge that my own memory and experiences are as constructed as any other woman's. As Donna Haraway reminds us, "Experience may also be *re*-constructed, re-membered, re-articulated" (*Simians* 113; see also Bruner, "Self-Making Narratives"; McAdams). The version here of my first birth story is somewhat different from the one I wrote in an email to my cousin April the day after the birth (there are far fewer expletives here, for example). This story is far more detailed than the thirty-two-word journal entry I wrote that day, which begins, "I had a baby!!" and ends with "Need sleep!" or the somewhat more varnished version I share orally; and it is far less detailed than the version I can imagine. Certain experiences—like pain, as Elaine Scarry has aptly demonstrated, but other bodily experiences, too—simply do not translate into words. The stories have changed as I've heard the impressions and memories of others who were present: my birth stories illustrate, then, the partial and problematic nature of stories of experience. They also illustrate, though, the ways such everyday rhetorics interact with and intervene in rhetorics of health and medicine. Like my mother's birth story, my stories can be interpreted in a variety of ways, each of which relies upon particular understandings of women, of people, and of science, medicine, and progress.

My stories, like my mother's, share a sense of the "nick of time," that *kairotic* significance of a lucky final-moment arrival, though for mine these have to do with a midwife's arrival at my home rather than my arrival at the hospital. My stories also illustrate how intuitive, bodily knowing can feel trickster-y—as with the coyote in many a southwestern tale, what seems at times to be "known" is not always as it seems. Like my mother's story, my stories provide anecdotal evidence of women's ability to labor naturally (though I don't believe *any* evidence to be applicable to all women's labors). My stories suggest a significant value in partner support, and they certainly testify to labor's unpredictability.

These stories of mine also illustrate the ways that educational knowledge and other women's assertions of feminist rhetorical agency can achieve effects beyond themselves. Other women's attempts to shape and collect their childbirth experience—to assert agency over their births—in turn shaped my experiences and helped me gain agency in childbirth. I gave birth at home because other women had experiences at home and shared their stories online. I gave birth at home because other women had experiences in hospitals and shared their stories online. I gave birth at home because midwives and scholars and physicians all wrote books supporting the notion that the vast majority of birth situations are unduly complicated by, rather than complemented by, hospitals. As this project illustrates, I am not the only woman whose birth choices have been affected by childbirth rhetorics such as online birth narratives, birth plans, and birth information shared by everyday women as much as or more than by information shared by officially sanctioned experts.

Each of my stories is important to me, as any woman's story is important to her as an individual, but beyond that, these stories, and interpretations of them, are significant for scholars seeking to understand the connections and effects of various kinds of rhetorics. Here I've examined how everyday rhetorics shared online, in concert with dominant discourses, affect contemporary, everyday American women (including myself) giving birth within a larger system of health and medicine, a system that we have only begun to study or understand rhetorically. Bringing these two elements together—the rhetorics of the everyday with rhetorics of health and medicine—is the primary contribution of this book.

Everyday women make use of feminist rhetorical agency, even if they do not consider themselves feminist, even if their rhetoric is dismissed by dominant discourses, and even if their assertions of agency fail to affect power relations in a given moment. Everyday women write. Everyday women write online. Everyday women write online and make things happen. Everyday women write online and make things happen for other individual, everyday women as well as for a broader culture. Everyday women write online and illustrate that broad cultural acceptance of a set of health care practices does not equate with that set of health care practices being the best, or the only, way to do things. Everyday women write online and open up new understandings and different possibilities for other everyday women. This book gives one glimpse into how.

APPENDIXES

NOTES

WORKS CITED

INDEX

APPENDIX A: SURVEY RECRUITMENT EMAIL

Subject line: Birth story research help?
(Later revised to: [Child's name]'s birth story/research help?)
Message contents:

Hi [mother's name, if known],

I read [child's name]'s birth story online and was very interested in it. Thank you for sharing your experience!

I am writing a dissertation on how and why women write about childbirth. I'm looking both at online birth stories and at birth plans. Your willingness to help others through sharing your birth story made me think you might be willing to help me with my research by responding to an online survey. The survey will take about 20 minutes, depending on how much you write. You can participate in the survey without using your name, if that would make you feel more comfortable.

The survey is available at: [web address]

I hope you'll take a few minutes to help me and other women learn more about childbirth and childbirth writing.

Feel free to respond to this email with any questions or comments, either before, after, or instead of completing the survey. Below you will find a consent form that describes the project and what you can expect if you choose to participate.

Thank you!
Sincerely,
Kim Hensley Owens

Childbirth Writing Survey
Consent Form
As a PhD candidate at [my university], I am researching how and why women write about childbirth. I am looking at birth plans and online birth stories to see what I can learn from them about childbirth practices and how writing may help women understand and deal with childbirth. This survey

asks women who have posted online birth stories to answer questions about their childbirth and writing experiences. This research will be used for my dissertation and may be used for conference presentations and published research in the future.

Participation is completely voluntary. You may refuse to participate or discontinue participation at any time. You may skip any questions you don't wish to answer.

Because this survey is going out only to those who have already made their stories public, there are no risks beyond those already encountered in everyday life. Anonymity will be protected where requested. This survey is not intended to benefit participants directly, but I hope and expect the information gathered to help other women to prepare for and deal with their childbirth experiences. No costs or payment are connected to this research project.

Your responses can be connected with your name or can be used anonymously. The second question of the survey asks for a name. If you prefer not to use your real name, you may create your own pseudonym. Question 21 asks if I may contact you by email to solicit a copy of your birth plan (if you wrote one). You should feel free to decline my request; doing so will have no bearing on any other aspect of your participation in this study.

If you have any questions about this research project, you may contact me, Kim Hensley Owens, PhD candidate in English, at: [my email address] or [phone number]. You may contact the IRB Office at: [IRB email address] or [phone number] for information about the rights of human research subjects.

The text of this consent form is included in my original email to you. You may print that information for your records. The copy of this consent form included with the survey serves as a reminder of the contents. The first question of the survey asks for your consent to participate based on this information.

If any question seems irrelevant or makes you uncomfortable, please feel free not to answer.

APPENDIX B: CHILDBIRTH WRITING SURVEY

1. I consent to participate in this research project. I understand that I may withdraw at any time by contacting Kim Hensley Owens at the email address or telephone number listed above.
2. Name (Please choose a pseudonym if you prefer not to use your real name. Indicate a pseudonym by placing a * before the name. Please make a note of any pseudonym you choose. If you choose to withdraw from the study at any time, you will need it.)
3. Email address (You may leave this blank if you wish to remain anonymous and/or prefer not to answer any follow-up questions.)

Writing Birth Stories

4. For which of your children did you write a birth story? (For multiple births, check the appropriate number—if your first birth you had twins, you would check "first and second") [options provided: first, second, third, fourth and/or subsequent births]
5. What year(s) did you give birth?
6. Why did you decide to share your story online? How did you find out about this option?
7. Who did you imagine as the audience for the stories? What effect did you intend your story to have on others? On yourself?
8. Before posting your story, did you write it in another form or revise it? Could you describe your writing process? Did you type or handwrite it first? Did you show it to anyone? Who? Why?
9. Do you read your own story or others' stories online? Why? How often? Has reading others' stories changed your perception of your story?
10. If you hadn't posted your story online, do you think you would have written it down? If so, where? (diary, letter, email, etc.) Why?
11. About how long after you gave birth did you first write your story? [options provided: within a week; within a month; a few months; a year or more]
12. About how long after you gave birth did you first post your story? [options provided: within a week; within a month; a few months; a year or more]

13. Please list the words or phrases that could complete this sentence: Writing/posting this story was _____ for me.

Childbirth Preparation

14. What did you do to prepare for/learn about childbirth? Whose advice did you follow? Did you join a pregnancy support group of any kind? Please describe if so.
15. What books or websites, if any, did you consult? Why? Would you recommend any of these to others? Why or why not?
16. How would you describe the role of insurance coverage in determining your childbirth options and experience?
17. What factors determined your childbirth preferences? Did reading online birth stories affect your expectations?

Birth Plans

18. Did you have a birth plan? If so, how did you find out what a birth plan was?
19. What models or templates did you work from to write your birth plan, if any? With whom did you write your birth plan, if anyone?
20. What did you expect your birth plan to accomplish? How closely were your expectations met? Do you see a different purpose for birth plans after having given birth?
21. If you still have a copy of your birth plan, would you be willing to share it with me for my research? (Please make sure your email address is included above if you say yes.)

Demographics

22. Current age and age(s) when you gave birth. Please indicate which birth(s) you posted narratives about.
23. Location (Please include your city and state and/or whether you are in an urban, rural, or suburban area.)
24. Race/Ethnicity [options provided: American Indian or Alaska Native; Asian; Black or African American; Latina; Multi-racial and or Multi-ethnic (please check all that apply); Native Hawaiian or Other Pacific Islander; White]
25. Religion/belief system
26. Parenting partnership, if any
27. Number of children you have given birth to

28. Occupation
29. Highest level of education [options provided: high school, some college, bachelor's degree, graduate degree]

Computer Use

30. Please check the places you use a computer and/or access the Internet: [options provided: home; work; library; school]
31. From where did you write and/or post a birth story? [options provided: home; work; library; school]
32. What are the three top reasons you go online, besides checking email?
33. How would you describe yourself as a computer user? [options provided: beginner; competent; expert]
34. How often do you use a computer/access the Internet? (Choose the answer that most closely matches your use) [options provided: multiple times a day; daily; weekly; monthly or less]
35. What kind of Internet access do you use most often? [options provided: dial-up/modem; DSL/broadband; cable modem; Ethernet; wireless; not sure]
36. Please share any other information you consider important or relevant—about your childbirth experience, writing about your experience, posting online, or anything else.

Thank you!

NOTES

Introduction: Writing Birth—Asserting Rhetorical Agency

1. The page remains live, with occasional updates about Ruth, who is perfectly healthy, and continues to accrue supportive messages.

2. See Amy Koerber's "Rhetorical Agency, Resistance, and the Disciplinary Rhetorics of Breastfeeding" on the ways individual agency and ideological force are "inextricably linked" (88).

3. As mentioned in the preface, I have left women's words as they posted them, including typos, to preserve their natural voices.

4. Women in this study have a variety of everyday vocations in addition to these three, including call center agent, historian, clerical worker, veterinary technician, self-employed worker, civil engineer, pharmacy technician, apprentice midwife and doula, writer, federal employee, housewife, math teacher, student, child-care provider, and freelance public relations consultant.

5. Chapter 1 provides more details about the history of childbirth.

6. A birth narrative on *Plomp.com*, for example, repeatedly refers to insurance: "we tried to get insurance to cover a midwife"; "I wanted a home birth but she only did hospital births because of insurance purposes"; "we lost our insurance" (Julie).

7. Any feminist scholar knows that the landmark text of women writing about women's health and medicine is *Our Bodies, Ourselves*, and rhetoricians are now coming to know more about the rhetorical contours of various versions of that text through Susan Wells's *Our Bodies, Ourselves and the Work of Writing. Writing Childbirth* both draws on and adds to the insights offered in Wells's book, as well as in other recent monographs in women's rhetorics and rhetorics of health and medicine, such as Elizabeth Britt's textured rhetorical analysis of infertility and mandated insurance, J. Blake Scott's rhetorical-cultural analysis of AIDS and an HIV clinic, and Judy Segal's rhetorical survey of various medical and health decision-making processes.

8. Cosslett's use of a hyphen is likely simply a British usage difference (she also writes "post-modern" where American scholars more commonly write "postmodern"), but the hyphen in "birth-stories" makes a visual and emotional linguistic connection between birth and story, a connection affirmed by the birth story writers in my study. Cosslett analyzes the two dominant views of childbirth: childbirth as a medical event attended by physicians, and read by

many feminists as disempowering, versus childbirth as a "natural" life event attended by midwives, and read by many feminists as empowering.

9. Also see Katherine Beckett's "Choosing Cesarean" for a detailed analysis of general rhetorical positions of these two dominant views.

10. These stories, unlike those on the ubiquitous "reality" television shows, provide women's own perspectives, in their own unedited words, on their own terms, appropriately for a book focusing on everyday women's writing. This is not to say, however, that women's written birth stories are never constrained or that reality show births have nothing to teach us (see Morris and McInerney).

11. Though not focused on childbirth per se, Marika Seigel's excellent new book, *The Rhetoric of Pregnancy*, is related in that it analyzes pregnancy manuals as forms of technical communication.

12. These websites align with what Philippa Spoel casts as "consumption model" websites—those offering anonymously exchanged information—rather than with "community model" websites, or those providing interactive interfaces and spaces to develop virtual relationships ("Communicating Values" 264). Although the sites and the women who post on them often seem to imagine more of a community model ethos (see chapter 4), the primary function of the sites is transactional rather than relationship-building.

13. Because I drew my participants from extant online birth narratives, I did not preselect or attempt to sample representative ages, races, ethnicities, classes, or sexual orientations. I anticipated more variety in respondent demographics than I found: all participants were white and married to a man, and nearly all participants identified as middle class and Christian. That my book is necessarily focused on this particular demographic suggests the need for future scholars to explore how race, class, ethnicity, gender, and sexual orientation affect women's childbirth rhetorics and the ways they interact with and create everyday rhetorics of health and medicine on- and offline.

14. In order to demonstrate how women might stumble upon these sites through searching for general birth information, I searched "birth," "childbirth," "birth stories" and "childbirth and labor" with three search engines, Google, Yahoo!, and AOL, and tracked the first page of results. (NB: AOL listed "sponsored links" before "web results," so while the web results were similar, readers would have had to scroll past that section, which did not include any of these five sites with any of the above search terms at the time of my 2005 search.) *Childbirth.org* appeared prominently (often first) in all four searches on each of these three search engines and thus was the most easily accessible. *BirthStories.com* and *TheLaborofLove.com* showed up with a "birth stories" search on all engines, and Google offered *Plomp.com* in this category as well. *UnassistedChildbirth.com* appeared with "childbirth" searches on both Google and AOL.

15. The survey (see appendixes A and B) focused on both writing and childbirth, delineating the function writing serves in preparing for and making sense of this complicated life event. To begin, I sent out thirty recruitment emails. I received over a dozen immediate responses: "mail daemon" messages. Nearly half of the posted email addresses were no longer functional. Beyond this setback, only one person from that initial batch completed the survey. My second and third rounds of recruitment emails met with similar fates until I hit upon a solution: I began using children's names in the subject line of the emails I sent. Instead of a subject line like "Birth story research help?," I tailored each request using subject lines like "Brayden's Birth Story—a research request?" Every birth story includes the child's name, even if the mother remains anonymous. Response rates improved dramatically.

1. Understanding Birth: Commonplaces of Modern American Childbirth Advice

1. On progress narratives, see Zerubavel, *Time Maps*. Also see Almond, Chodorow, and Pearce.

2. The data is further defined for black and white women (with no other racial data offered): white women's maternal mortality is 7.6 per 100,000, or 0.0076 percent, and black women's maternal mortality rate is significantly higher, though still a fraction of historical rates, at 30.5 per 100,000, or 0.0305 percent (Hoyert et al.).

3. See Dye; Loudon; Mintz; and Tague.

4. Based on what follows this question, I read Iovine's phrase "poor women" to mean not women of a low socioeconomic status but women deserving of our pity. Also, despite persistent beliefs to the contrary, maternal mortality, unlike infant mortality, has historically been higher in women of higher, rather than lower, socioeconomic status. See Loudon.

5. See, for example, Tague; and Arriaza, Allison, and Gerszten. Childbirth-related complications reached a level of 14 percent of women between twelve and forty-five in a sample of pre-Columbian Andean mummies, the highest rate of maternal mortality I found. Tague reviews literature that suggests improper or unsanitary methods of delivery were to blame.

6. Drawing on women's everyday texts such as diaries and letters, Judith Leavitt finds that colonial women's fears of dying dominated their thoughts and plans before birth. She explains that women "armed themselves against the fearful aspects of childbirth by seeking the support of other women who had passed through the experience successfully" (*Brought to Bed* 7).

7. Describing maternal mortality for a general audience online, historian Steven Mintz offers this interpretation of historical maternal mortality data:

> During the seventeenth and eighteenth centuries, between 1 percent and 1.5 percent of all births ended in the mother's death as a result of exhaustion, dehydration, infection, hemorrhage, or convulsions. Since the typical mother gave birth to between five and eight children, her lifetime chances of dying in childbirth ran as high as 1 in 8. *This meant that if a woman had eight female friends, it was likely that one might die in childbirth.* (my emphasis)

Mintz's explanatory conclusion here seems an overstatement, given that he relies on both upper ends of statistical likelihood for his odds, without a corresponding use of both lower ends. Relying on both lower ends provides a ratio closer to one in twenty, or 0.05 percent—still an unpalatable figure, but one with a rather different effect than one in eight, or 12.5 percent.

8. See Wertz and Wertz, who rely upon such primary sources as colonial midwife Martha Ballard's diary (a source later contextualized and analyzed by historian Laurel Thatcher in *A Midwife's Tale*).

9. Historically, "midwife" referred to women trained through apprenticeship. Today there are two distinct paths to "midwife." A certified professional midwife (CPM) is a lay (also called direct-entry, or traditional) midwife, who trains with apprenticeship and schooling; a certified nurse midwife (CNM) is a nurse who completes additional midwifery coursework. CPMs usually practice outside of the medical hierarchy and have no hospital privileges (though it is best for all if an obstetrician will provide back-up services in case of hospital transfer). CNMs tend to practice in hospitals and are often subject to medical hierarchies. In some states CNMs can legally perform home births. See Cassidy; Gaskin, *Spiritual Midwifery*; Lay; and Taylor.

10. Readers might wonder what the role of husbands/fathers has been over time. Judith Leavitt, in *Make Room for Daddy*, shows that after centuries of exclusion from childbirth (an exclusion that continued when women began birthing in hospitals), men gained entry to hospital delivery rooms by the 1970s. Fathers' access did not initially extend to operating rooms, however. In fact, Leavitt's book reveals absoluteness of obstetrical staffs' control over hospital labor and couples' corresponding lack of agency over even such details as a partner's presence. By the 1980s fathers were permitted to attend all elements of labor and delivery (281). While the evolution of men's presence in US hospital births suggests inclusion and equality, Leavitt finds that this "seemingly radical change," a change the women's movement supported, ultimately "*reinforced physicians' authority and family gender hierarchies*" (287; emphasis in original).

11. Thomas Kuhn says textbooks are "systematically misleading" with regard to providing authentic historical information, because textbooks aim to communicate a contemporary society's syntax and science (137).

12. See Weerasekera for an example of ways modern physicians seek to minimize such injuries.

13. Individual births and individual care providers are always unique: when I speak of tendencies and dominant acts or choices made by particular types of care providers, I am speaking generally, based on my findings and widespread perceptions, but individuals defy expectations in all directions. Certainly physicians can provide emotional support and/or technology-free births and midwives can provide emotionally unsupportive births and/or (over)rely on technology and interventions.

14. For a detailed examination of electronic fetal monitoring, see Cartwright.

15. For a cogent material rhetoric analysis of freestanding birth centers as sites that provide women increased agency in countering hegemonic medical models of childbirth, see Schuster.

2. Inventing Birth: Rhetorics of Control and Resistance

1. Do Not Resuscitate orders are another instance of patient-doctor written communication, albeit one with a legal force (or an anticipated legal force—see Keränen) that birth plans do not have. See chapter 3 for more discussion of DNRs.

2. Here I am invoking, as mentioned in the introduction, Martin Nystrand and John Duffy's definition of rhetoric as "the ways that individuals and groups use language to constitute their social realities, and as a medium for creating, managing, or resisting ideological meanings" (ix).

3. The Google Labs Ngram Viewer is an online search tool developed by researchers at Harvard University's Cultural Observatory. The ngram allows users to search "over 5.2 million books" to determine the frequency of a word or phrase's appearance (Michel et al., "Quantitative Analysis").

4. For an easily digestible, research-supported narrative describing what I'm calling the "typical American birth," see Taylor's *Giving Birth*. For meticulously researched historical data, including statistical analyses, see Rooks. See Leavitt, *Brought to Bed*, for a thorough history of childbirth and women's efforts to control it. Also see Ulrich on colonial midwifery practices. For a rhetorical analysis of midwifery as it contrasts with this medical model, see Lay's *Rhetoric of Midwifery*. Mitford writes of American birthing practices in exposé style. For a detailed analysis of obstetric beliefs and practices, see Goer. Treichler offers a rich analysis of the "meaning" of childbirth in America. Wolf provides a personal account of birth in the late 1990s interwoven with research.

5. Hospital births differ by attendants, and there is a difference between physician-attended and certified nurse midwife–attended births, but although a 2011 study (Osterman and Martin) confirms that women giving birth vaginally

and attended by CNMs in 2008 received epidurals (one example of pain medication) less often than women attended by physicians, epidural use is nonetheless common. Over 60 percent of women in the study whose babies were delivered by physicians received epidurals, while 49.8 percent of women attended by CNMs received epidurals. Since a significant majority of women are attended in labor by physicians, significantly more than half of all hospital births include epidural anesthesia. Other medications are also employed, both on their own and in addition to epidurals, in hospital settings.

6. Lay offers a detailed description of these multiple knowledges brought to bear on childbirth in *Rhetoric of Midwifery.*

7. Methods for determining a woman's due date range from counting 280 days (forty weeks) from the first day of the last normal menstrual period to estimating gestational age through ultrasound. Henci Goer explains that (white, middle-class) women bearing their first child average 288 days, with subsequent pregnancies lasting 283 days, and that the margin of error for pregnancy dating via ultrasound, while only 5 days in the first trimester, increases to a whopping 22 days in the third (180). She adds that black women have, on average, 8.5 fewer days of gestational time than white women; she includes no other racial/ethnic data.

8. It is easy to see how women used to controlling (*chronos*-based) time in their everyday lives might opt to schedule a C-section (typically no more than a thirty-minute procedure, usually significantly faster) at their convenience, rather than wait for a possibly inconvenient, hours- or days-long labor (*kairos*-based time).

9. It should be noted that material constraints such as room and equipment availability also contribute. A hospital's allocation of resources also plays a role in the way time is understood and valued. Thus, materiality affects concepts of time, which in turn affect materiality.

10. Nipple stimulation releases oxytocin, the hormone connected to both sexual arousal and the onset of labor. Pitocin is a synthetic version of oxytocin, which stimulates and speeds up contractions. Pitocin lacks the multifaceted effects of natural oxytocin; the latter can also bring pleasure and a sense of calm.

11. While not a part of my corpus of online texts, an obstetrician's "birth plan" (posted by one of his patients), addressed to his patients, illustrates the ways the concept of birth plan has been taken up far beyond women's desires. He makes unequivocal statements about what he will and will not do for women in labor, such as "I do not accept birth plans"; "I do not accept the Bradley Birth Plan"; "IV access during labor is mandatory"; "Continuous monitoring . . . is mandatory"; and "I perform all vaginal deliveries on a standard labor and delivery bed. . . . This is the most comfortable position for you. It also

provides the maximum space in your pelvis" ("OB's Birth Plan"). While the tone of the "birth plan" is exceptionally condescending and a cruel parody of women's birth plans, it is that last quotation that stands out, given that it is patently false (Wagner 40–41.)

12. Certainly many women appreciate this omission, preferring not to consider unpleasant outcomes, but I suspect, with Layne, that such omissions, whether in templates or by women choosing not to read information about miscarriage or stillbirth, exacerbate the emotional and intellectual challenges of such outcomes, and possibly the physical as well.

13. See Anne Fadiman's *The Spirit Catches You and You Fall Down*.

14. Over the course of this study, *Birthplan.com* changed how users access the online birth planner. The 2005 version appeared with a click. By 2011, users were required to create a username and password, enter an imaged security code, agree to an updated privacy policy and a "new Terms of Use" policy, and check boxes (or rather, uncheck boxes, as they are checked by default) for receiving, for example, "occasional updates, special offers, and other information from Disney Family." The 2011 version, Disney-ified, has a much stronger emphasis on consumerism and on the copyright protection of the site hosting the information. It seems particularly disappointing that a tool designed for a woman to create a birth plan—a document explicitly intended for use at a hospital or birthing center—is labeled with the boilerplate legal terminology "for your personal, noncommercial home use only."

15. For an analysis of the intersections between Internet health users' expertise versus that of physicians, see Hensley Owens, "Rhetorics of E-Health and Information Age Medicine."

16. The checklist options in the "Our birth plan" template that may not be readable in Figure 2.4 include "remain mobile during labor"; "no shave prep"; "no routine IV's; "no enema (either at home or on site)"; "to urinate on my own"; "my partner ALWAYS present"; "to have low level lighting in the room"; "to eat and drink during labor"; "only intermittent fetal monitoring"; "spontaneous rupture of membranes"; "pain relief/epidural if I ask"; "to use various positions"; "to use aroma therapy"; "to have massages"; "to listen to music"; "to NOT have pitocin." Under "Vaginal Delivery options" the portion of the list visible in Figure 2.4 includes "no episiotomy"; "perineal massage"; "my partner to cut the cord"; "my partner to bath [*sic*] the baby after birth."

3. Confronting Birth: Rhetorical Disability and Five Women's Birth Plans

1. Perhaps because women expressing desires vocally during birth are often not taken seriously (Dwinell 14).

2. Thirty-four women responded to the survey, seventeen of whom had written birth plans. Most women had not kept their birth plans, seeing no use for them after the birth.

3. Anecdotally, I've heard stories about birth plans being ripped up, ignored, and/or laughed at. My favorite of these stories is one where a friend handed her birth plan to the nurse at the start of her labor and the nurse waved it away, shaking her head and repeating, "Those things are voodoo." The nurse turned out to be quite supportive of my friend's desires, but not at all receptive to the written birth plan.

4. Because the survey gave women the option of remaining anonymous or using a pseudonym, which several women did, I was not always able to match women's birth plans with their online birth narratives.

5. Former obstetrician Judith Brysk opines that her patients often didn't understand the consequences of their birth plan choices; she respected patients' wishes but expected them to trust her knowledge and training above all. Also, see Ellen Barton, who describes the challenges of patients and physicians negotiating expertise. Barton complicates the concept of expertise, showing that it belongs exclusively to neither physicians nor patients but rather must be constantly negotiated. The rhetorical failure of many women's birth plans suggests hospital birth as a context where such negotiations seem to favor physician expertise.

6. As with most landmark studies, theirs has its share of critics along with its adherents. For a comprehensive review of critiques of Brown and Levinson's theory, and an alternate view of politeness, see Watts, *Politeness*. Christine Christie also provides a critique of Brown and Levinson's too-ready dismissal of potential gender differences in politeness in *Gender and Language*.

7. Brown and Levinson focus on oral communication, but the theory applies equally well to writing.

8. While DNRs, living wills, and other forms of advance care directives are perceived to be legally binding documents in ways birth plans are not, such end-of-life requests are not always honored, either. Recently researchers have begun suggesting that advance care planning focus less on predetermined, specific directives and more on shaping physicians' responses to the emotional needs of families and patients. See Tulsky, "Beyond Advance Directives."

9. And so, birth planning may need to evolve as advance care directives are suggested to, to help physicians better consider their patients' emotional and medical needs based on discussions with the woman and her partner, prior to and during birth (see Tulsky, "Beyond Advance Directives").

4. Hosting Birth: Birth and Birth Stories over Time and Online

1. As pointed out in the introduction, the websites are *BirthStories.com*, *Childbirth.org*, *TheLaborofLove.com*, *Plomp.com*, and *UnassistedChildbirth.*

com, which demonstrate the breadth of options readily available online in the early twenty-first century. In 2004–5, each site came up in the first page of Yahoo, AOL, and Google searches for "birth stories." The women I surveyed relied on one or more of these five sites to post their birth narratives and/or to read stories. In 2009, *Plomp.com* went offline; because it was available to the women I surveyed and hosted several stories included in my archive, the site remains in my study. I analyze the *kairotic* context of each site as it existed at the time of my survey, as well as describe how the sites have changed and continue to evolve.

2. Leavitt in *Brought to Bed* reports fertility rates (number of live births per woman) for American white married women to have been 7.04 in 1800 and 3.65 in 1900. She reports fertility rates for black women in 1900 to be over 5. The 2000 US census report indicates fertility rates for different races (regardless of marital status): women's overall fertility rate (ages fifteen to forty-four), 1.22 (much lower than the 2.2 that circulates popularly); white women, 1.21; white non-Hispanic women, 1.15; black women, 1.35; Asian and Pacific Islander women, 0.97; Hispanic women, 1.51. (The census numbers were originally presented as per 1,000 women; I adjusted the numbers to reflect rates for individuals for ease of comparison with Leavitt's data.)

3. See also Ulrich, *A Midwife's Tale*. This colonial-era diary of a midwife corroborates social childbirth practices.

4. The practice of having laywomen attend births is increasing, perhaps because numerous studies have demonstrated significant benefits for women both during labor and postpartum. A review of twelve such studies recommends that "every woman [have] access to continuous emotional and physical support during labor" (Scott, Klaus, and Klaus 1257). Such female lay support can be provided by doulas (a Greek term whose meaning has shifted from "woman servant" to "woman who provides labor support"), who are becoming increasingly available for hospital births around the country. See, for example, Wilgoren, "'Mothering the Mother.'"

5. Prior to the 1970s, there were very few books about pregnancy and childbirth for laywomen. As Susan Wells explains in *Our Bodies, Ourselves and the Work of Writing*, one goal of the authors of *Our Bodies, Ourselves* was to provide women with health and medical information in women's own words.

6. Additionally, some women's stories never appeared on the sites where they were sent. One respondent laments,

> I had submitted a second narrative about my son Jaron's birth and never knew whether it had been posted or not. The last time I had checked was a year after I had posted it, and it still wasn't there. . . .

> I got some responses as to something about being backlogged and thought that was kind of a lame excuse . . . so I never returned to post my third baby's birth or to check on the status of my other stories. (Shannon, survey)

7. This graphic appeared on the website from May 2000 until a complete redesign of the site in November 2005. Screen captures of the pages including the graphic are available online through the *Internet Archive Wayback Machine*. *BirthStories.com* now routes to *Babble.com*, owned by Disney Enterprises, which declined to grant permission to use the image of the graphic in this book.

8. Disney also declined permission to use any of those images here.

9. "Unassisted childbirth" can be interpreted in somewhat different ways by different women: for some it means birthing entirely alone; for others it means other people may be present but not physically involved. Husbands in these stories often appear as photographers.

5. Sharing Birth: Catharsis, Commentary, and Testimonial in Online Birth Stories

1. Narration "is coherence seeking and coherence guarding, eschewing dissonance and contradiction through highly developed psychic procedures" (Bruner, "Self-Making Narratives" 214).

2. Likely worth mentioning is that with the advent of Web 2.0 spaces from Tumblr to Twitter, more and more women can and do post online—and some certainly harness those spaces as sites for feminist power. Though not all women's posts make feminist claims, either explicitly or implicitly, posts on those sites often illustrate the ways the personal and the political are intertwined. Examining Tumblr and Twitter posts about childbirth is out of the scope of this study but would be another way of accessing women's publicly shared stories (or microstories) about childbirth.

3. Because some women left this question blank and many women gave more than one response, numbers here do not correspond to the number of survey respondents.

4. Four of the sixteen "transformative" responses are not accounted for. Two women who experienced benefits from writing wrote about multiple births with drastically different outcomes and perceptions of their own control over them; from the data available it remains unclear whether the writing helped only with particular births, traumatic or otherwise, or with all of them. The two remaining women for whom writing proved cathartic did not provide the identification information that would enable me to compare their birth narratives and survey responses.

5. Walking can be of enormous benefit in reducing labor's length and intensity, as Sandy was seemingly aware from her reading. Walking is difficult in most hospital birth settings, however, and with a monitor attached, walking is not an option.

6. The abbreviation "dh" for "dear husband" is common online. It appears frequently in online birth narratives and on the sites where they appear. Despite loving association of the word "dear," or perhaps because "dear" can be employed sarcastically, as "dh" often is in the narratives, the term also suggests a certain distancing.

7. Ischial spines are bony protrusions in the pelvic bones. Physicians and midwives use the spines to gauge a baby's progress, or "station." When the presenting portion of the baby is above the spines, the station is recorded as a negative number; when it is even with the spines, the baby is at station zero; and when it passes the spines, the station is recorded as a positive number (in centimeters) (Cunningham et al. 426). When a baby is at +3, delivery is usually imminent.

Epilogue: Experiencing Birth

1. To "strip the membranes," a birth attendant uses a finger inserted in the cervix to separate the amniotic sac from the uterine wall.

2. I know some readers will assume that I believe everyone should have home births, so I want to be clear that while I advocate women having that *option*, legally and easily and cost effectively, I do not advocate home birth for all women any more than I would advocate general anesthesia C-sections for all women. If this book demonstrates anything about women and choice, I hope it is that women need to be able to make their own choices, rhetorically and materially.

3. The provider and "procedure" were preapproved at 100 percent coverage after several rounds of phone conversations with myriad representatives from the insurance company, all of which began with what they referred to as a required portion of the "application," a "date for the procedure." Since I was planning to *give birth*, a *kairotic* event, providing an advance date and calling it a "procedure" rankled. Despite that advance approval, I was billed for 20 percent of the midwife's fee. Several more phone calls and a letter resulted in a retraction of that bill but with significant language about the 100 percent payment being a result of errors made and reminders that any future home births would not be covered at 100 percent.

WORKS CITED

"Achievements in Public Health, 1900–1999: Healthier Mothers and Babies." *Morbidity and Mortality Weekly Report* 48.38 (1999): 849–58. Centers for Disease Control and Prevention. 1 Oct. 1999. Web. 15 Mar. 2006.

Adams, Alice E. *Reproducing the Womb: Images of Childbirth in Science, Feminist Theory, and Literature*. Ithaca, NY: Cornell UP, 1994. Print.

Allende, Isabel. *Paula*. New York: HarperCollins, 1995. Print.

Almond, Gabriel A., Marvin Chodorow, and Roy Harvey Pearce, eds. *Progress and Its Discontents*. Berkeley: U of California P, 1977. Print.

Ame. "Birth Story of Lillian Marie Smith." *Plomp.com*. n.d. Web. 12 Mar. 2005.

Amy. "My Vbac Homebirth." *TheLaborofLove.com*. n.d. Web. 18 Feb. 2009.

Anderson, G. C., E. Moore, J. Hepworth, and N. Bergman. "Early Skin-to-Skin Contact for Mothers and Their Healthy Newborn Infants." *Cochrane Database of Systematic Reviews* 2 (2003): PubMed. 12804473. Web. 5 May 2006.

Anna. "Birth Story of Karina." *Plomp.com*. 9 Dec. 2004. Web. 10 Feb. 2006.

Arms, Suzanne. *Immaculate Deception: A New Look at Women and Childbirth in America*. Boston: Houghton Mifflin, 1975. Print.

———. *Immaculate Deception II: Myth, Magic, and Birth*. Berkeley: Celestial Arts, 1996. Print.

Arney, William Ray. *Power and the Profession of Obstetrics*. Chicago: U of Chicago P, 1982. Print.

Arriaza, Bernardo, Marvin Allison, and Enrique Gerszten. "Maternal Mortality in Pre-Columbian Indians of Arica, Chile." *American Journal of Physical Anthropology* 77 (1988): 35–41. Web. 14 Feb. 2009.

Aubry, Richard. "Foreword: A Word from the Doctor." *What to Expect When You're Expecting*. Ed. Arlene Eisenberg, Heidi E. Murkoff, and Sandee E. Hathaway. New York: Workman, 2002. xx–xvi. Print.

Autumn. "Five Hours of Pushing = Perfect Princess." *BirthStories.com*. n.d. Web. 26 Jan. 2006.

Barton, Ellen L. "The Social Work of Diagnosis: Evidence for Judgments of Competence and Incompetence." *Constructing (in)Competence: Disabling Evaluations in Clinical and Social Interaction*. Ed. Dana Kovarsky, Judith Duchan, and Madeline Maxwell. Hillsdale: Lawrence Erlbaum, 1999. 257–90. Print.

Baxley, Elizabeth G., and Robert W. Gabbo. "Shoulder Dystocia." *American Family Physician* 69.7 (2004): 1707–14. Print.

Bazerman, Charles, and Paul Prior, eds. *What Writing Is and How It Does It.* Mahwah, NJ: Lawrence Erlbaum, 2004. Print.

Beatrice. "Dora's Birth Story." *Bornfree.com.* n.d. Web. 5 Mar. 2005.

Beckett, Katherine. "Choosing Cesarean: Feminism and the Politics of Childbirth in the United States." *Feminist Theory* 6.3 (2005): 251–75. Print.

Bérubé, Michael. *Life as We Know It: A Father, a Family, and an Exceptional Child.* New York: Vintage, 1996. Print.

Beth. "Birth Story of Brendan David Hoover." *TheLaborofLove.com.* n.d. Web. 5 Dec. 2005.

Birke, Lynda. *Feminism and the Biological Body.* New Brunswick, NJ: Rutgers UP, 2000. Print.

Birmingham, Elizabeth. "Another Fine Mess: The Pregnant Body and the Discipline of the Line." *WOE: Writing on the Edge* 14.2 (2004): 95–109. Print.

"Birth Plan: Create Your Birth Plan." *Pregnancy Today. BirthStories.com.* n.d. Web. 26 May 2011.

"Birth Plans." *Obgyn.net.* Listserv. June 1997. Web. 21 July 2005.

"BirthStories.com." *Internet Archive Wayback Machine.* 23 Nov. 2004. Web. 17 Nov. 2005.

"Birth Stories: Submit Your Birth Story." *Pregnancy Today. BirthStories.com.* n.d. Web. 13 Jan. 2011.

Bohjalian, Chris. *Midwives.* New York: Harmony, 1997. Print.

Bolter, Jay David, and Richard Grusin. "Remediation." *Configurations* 4.2 (1996): 311–58. Print.

Borst, Charlotte. *Catching Babies: The Professionalization of Childbirth, 1870–1920.* Cambridge, MA: Harvard UP, 1995. Print.

Boston Women's Health Book Collective. *Our Bodies, Ourselves: A Book by and for Women.* 1971. New York: Simon and Schuster, 1976. Print.

Bourdieu, Pierre. *The Logic of Practice.* Trans. Richard Nice. Stanford: Stanford UP, 1990. Print.

Britt, Elizabeth C. *Conceiving Normalcy: Rhetoric, Law, and the Double Binds of Infertility.* Tuscaloosa: U of Alabama P, 2001. Print.

Brodkey, Linda. *Academic Writing as Social Practice.* Philadelphia: Temple UP, 1987. Print.

———. *Writing Permitted in Designated Areas Only.* Minneapolis: U of Minnesota P, 1996. Print.

Brodsky, Phyllis. *The Control of Childbirth: Women versus Medicine through the Ages.* London: McFarland, 2008. Print.

Brown, Penelope, and Stephen C. Levinson. *Politeness: Some Universals in Language Use.* 1978. Cambridge: Cambridge UP, 1987. Print.

Brueggemann, Brenda Jo. "Still-Life." *Ethics and Representations in Qualitative Studies of Literacy.* Ed. Peter Mortensen and Gesa Kirsch. Urbana: NCTE, 1996. 17–34. Print.

Bruner, Jerome S. *Making Stories: Law, Literature, Life.* Cambridge, MA: Harvard UP, 2003. Print.

———. "The 'Remembered' Self." *The Remembering Self: Construction and Accuracy in the Self-Narrative.* Ed. Ulrich Neisser and Robyn Fivush. Cambridge: Cambridge UP, 1994. 41–54. Print.

———. "Self-Making Narratives." *Autobiographical Memory and the Construction of Narrative Self: Developmental and Cultural Perspectives.* Ed. Robyn Fivush and Catherine A. Haden. Mahwah, NJ: Lawrence Erlbaum, 2003. 209–26. Print.

Brysk, Judith. Personal interview. 4 Aug. 2005.

Bunkers, Suzanne L., and Cynthia Anne Huff. *Inscribing the Daily: Critical Essays on Women's Diaries.* Amherst: U of Massachusetts P, 1996. Print.

Burke, Kenneth. *Language as Symbolic Action; Essays on Life, Literature, and Method.* Berkeley: U of California P, 1966. Print.

———. *Permanence and Change: An Anatomy of Purpose.* 3rd ed., with a new afterword. Berkeley: U of California P, 1984. Print.

Butler, Judith. *Gender Trouble: Feminism and the Subversion of Identity.* Thinking Gender. New York: Routledge, 1990. Print.

Campbell, Karlyn Kohrs. "Agency: Promiscuous and Protean." *Communication and Critical/Cultural Studies* 2.1 (2005): 1–19. Print. doi:10.1080/1479142042000332134.

Cartwright, Elizabeth. "Electronic Fetal Monitoring and Biomedically Constructed Birth." *Cyborg Babies: From Techno-Sex to Techno-Tots.* Ed. Robbie Davis-Floyd and Joseph Dumit. New York: Routledge, 1998. 240–54. Print.

Cassidy, Tina. *Birth: The Surprising History of How We Are Born.* New York: Grove Press, 2006. Print.

"Catharsis." 1989. *Oxford English Dictionary Online.* Web. 15 Mar. 2007.

Catherine. "Birth Story of Cynthia Cailey." *Plomp.com.* n.d. Web. Dec. 2005.

Chassie. "Birth Story of Jayda." *Plomp.com.* 30 Dec. 2004. Web. 15 Nov. 2006.

Chen, Pi-chao, and Bizhao Zhen. *Population and Health Policy in the People's Republic of China.* Interdisciplinary Communications Program, Smithsonian Institute. 1976. Web. 18 May 2011.

Cheyney, Melissa. *In Transition: A Biocultural Analysis of Homebirth Midwifery in the United States.* Diss. University of Oregon, 2005. Print.

Christie, Christine. *Gender and Language: Towards a Feminist Pragmatics.* Edinburgh: Edinburgh UP, 2000. Print.

Cintron, Ralph. "'Gates Locked' and the Violence of Fixation." *Towards a Rhetoric of Everyday Life: New Directions in Research on Writing, Text, and Discourse.* Ed. Martin Nystrand and John Duffy. Madison: U of Wisconsin P, 2003. 5–37. Print.

Connors, Robert. "Dreams and Play." *Methods and Methodology in Composition Research.* Ed. Gesa Kirsch and Patricia Sullivan. Carbondale: Southern Illinois UP, 1992. 15–36. Print.

Corey. "Finding Truth." *Bornfree.com.* n.d. Web. 6 July 2005.

Cosslett, Tess. *Women Writing Childbirth: Modern Discourses of Motherhood.* Manchester: Manchester UP, 1994. Print.

Crowley, Sharon. *Composition in the University: Historical and Polemical Essays.* Pittsburgh: U of Pittsburgh P, 1998. Print.

Cuddy, Sabrina. "Birth Planning." *Fensende.com.* n.d. Web. 20 July 2005.

Cunningham, F. Gary, et al. *Williams Obstetrics.* 22nd ed. New York: McGraw Hill, 2005. Print.

Curtin, S. C., and M. M. Park. "Trends in the Attendant, Place, and Timing of Births, and in the Use of Obstetric Interventions: United States, 1989–97." *National Vital Statistics Reports, Centers for Disease Control and Prevention, National Center for Health Statistics National Vital Statistics System* 47.27 (1999): 1–16. Web. 4 Aug. 2008.

Cutter, Irving S., and Henry R. Viets. *A Short History of Midwifery.* Philadelphia: W. B. Saunders, 1964. Print.

Cynthia. "Birth Story of Bridges." *Plomp.com.* n.d. Web. 26 Jan. 2006.

Danielle. "The Birth of Louise Rose." *TheLaborofLove.com.* n.d. Web. 15 May 2006.

Davis-Floyd, Robbie. *Birth as an American Rite of Passage.* Berkeley: U of California P, 1992. Print.

Davis-Floyd, Robbie, and Joseph Dumit. "From Technobirth to Cyborg Babies." *Cyborg Babies: From Techno-Sex to Techno-Tots.* Ed. Robbie Davis-Floyd and Joseph Dumit. New York: Routledge, 1998. 255–84. Print.

"Deaths: Final Data for 2003." *NCHA Health E-Stat.* Centers for Disease Control and Prevention. 7 Jan. 2010. Web. 2 Feb. 2012.

De Certeau, Michel. *The Practice of Everyday Life.* Berkeley: U of California P, 1984. Print.

Devitt, Amy J. *Writing Genres.* Carbondale: Southern Illinois UP, 2004. Print.

Dickens, Charles. *Oliver Twist.* London: Penguin, 1871. Print.

Dickson, Barbara. "Reading Maternity Materially." *Rhetorical Bodies.* Ed. Jack Selzer and Sharon Crowley. Madison: U of Wisconsin P, 1999. 297–313. Print.

Duffy, John. "Other Gods and Countries: The Rhetoric of Literacy." *Towards a Rhetoric of Everyday Life: New Directions in Research on Writing, Text, and*

Discourse. Ed. Martin Nystrand and John Duffy. Madison: U of Wisconsin P, 2003. 38–57. Print.

Dumit, Joseph, and Sylvia Sensiper. "Living with the 'Truths' of DES: Toward an Anthropology of Facts." *Cyborg Babies: From Techno-Sex to Techno-Tots*. Ed. Robbie Davis-Floyd and Joseph Dumit. New York: Routledge, 1998. 212–39. Print.

Dwinell, Jane, RN. *Birth Stories: Mystery, Power, and Creation*. Westport, CT: Bergin and Garvey, 1992. Print.

Dye, Nancy Schrom. "History of Childbirth in America." *Signs* 6.1 (1980): 97–108. Print.

Eakin, Paul John. *How Our Lives Become Stories: Making Selves*. Ithaca: Cornell UP, 1999. Print.

Eastman, Nicholas J., and Louis M. Hellman. *Williams Obstetrics*. 13th ed. New York: Appleton-Century-Crofts, 1966. Print.

Ecker, Jeffery L., and Fredric D. Frigoletto Jr. "Cesarean Delivery and the Risk-Benefit Calculus." *New England Journal of Medicine* 365.9 (2007): 885–88. Print.

Edwards, Margot, and Mary Waldorf. *Reclaiming Birth: History and Heroines of American Childbirth Reform*. Trumansburg, NY: Crossing, 1984. Print.

Ehrenreich, Barbara, and Dierdre English. *Witches, Midwives, and Nurses: A History of Women Healers*. New York: Feminist Press at SUNY, 1973. Print.

Ellis, Carolyn, and Arthur P. Bochner. "Autoethnography, Personal Narrative, Reflexivity." *Handbook of Qualitative Research*. Ed. Norman K. Denzin and Yvonna S. Lincoln. 2nd ed. Thousand Oaks, CA: Sage, 2000. 733–68. Print.

England, Pam, and Rob Horowitz. *Birthing from Within: An Extra-Ordinary Guide to Childbirth Preparation*. Albuquerque, NM: Partera, 1998. Print.

Epstein, Abby, dir. *The Business of Being Born*. New Line Home Entertainment and Red Envelope Entertainment. 2008. DVD.

Fadiman, Anne. *The Spirit Catches You and You Fall Down: A Hmong Child, Her American Doctors, and the Collision of Two Cultures*. New York: Farrar, Straus and Giroux, 1997. Print.

Fahnestock, Jeanne. "Accommodating Science: The Rhetorical Life of Scientific Facts." *Written Communication* 15.3 (1986): 275–96. Print.

Flannery, Kathryn Thomas. *Feminist Literacies, 1968–75*. Urbana: U of Illinois P, 2005. Print.

Fletcher, Ruth. "Reproductive Consumption." *Feminist Theory* 7.1 (2006): 27–47. Print.

Foucault, Michel. *Discipline and Punish: The Birth of the Prison*. Trans. Alan Sheridan. 1975. New York: Vintage, 1997. Print.

———. *The History of Sexuality*. Vol. 1. New York: Pantheon, 1978. Print.

———. "Technologies of the Self." *Technologies of the Self: A Seminar with Michel Foucault*. Ed. Luther H. Martin, Huck Gutman, and Patrick H. Hutton. Amherst: U of Massachusetts P, 1988. 16–49. Print.

Fox, Susannah. "Online Health Search 2006." *Pew Internet & American Life Project*. 29 Oct. 2006. Web. 2 Mar. 2012.

Gabriela. "A Generous Orgasm." *UnassistedChildbirth.com*. n.d. Web. 30 May 2006.

García Márquez, Gabriel. *One Hundred Years of Solitude*. Trans. Gregory Rabassa. New York: Harper and Row, 1970. Print.

Gaskin, Ina May. *Ina May's Guide to Childbirth*. New York: Bantam, 2003. Print.

———. *Spiritual Midwifery*. Summertown, TN: Book Publishing Co., 1978. Print.

Gawande, Atul. "The Score: How Childbirth Went Industrial." *NewYorker.com*. 9 Oct. 2006. Web. 19 Feb. 2007.

Geertz, Clifford. "Thick Description: Toward an Interpretive Theory of Culture." New York: Basic, 1973. 3–30. Print.

Goer, Henci. *Obstetric Myths versus Research Realities: A Guide to Medical Literature*. Westport, CT: Bergin and Garvey, 1995. Print.

Grant-Davie, Keith. "Coding Data." *Methods and Methodology in Composition Research*. Ed. Gesa Kirsch and Patricia Sullivan. Carbondale: Southern Illinois UP, 1992. 270–86. Print.

Grosz, Elizabeth A. *Volatile Bodies: Toward a Corporeal Feminism*. Bloomington: Indiana UP, 1994. Print.

Haraway, Donna J. *The Haraway Reader*. New York: Routledge, 2004. Print.

———. *Simians, Cyborgs, and Women: The Reinvention of Nature*. New York: Routledge, 1991. Print.

Harris, Judith. *Signifying Pain: Constructing and Healing the Self through Writing*. Albany: SUNY P, 2003. Print.

Harrison, Michelle, MD. *A Woman in Residence*. New York: Random House, 1982. Print.

Hauser, Gerard A. *Vernacular Voices: The Rhetoric of Publics and Public Spheres*. Columbia: U of South Carolina P, 1999. Print.

Hawhee, Debra. *Bodily Arts: Rhetoric and Athletics in Ancient Greece*. Austin: U of Texas P, 2004. Print.

Hawisher, Gail E., and Patricia Sullivan. "Women on the Networks: Searching for E-Spaces of Their Own." *Feminism and Composition Studies: In Other Words*. Ed. Susan C. Jarratt and Lynn Worsham. New York: MLA, 1998. 172–97. Print.

Hayles, N. Katherine. *How We Became Posthuman: Virtual Bodies in Cybernetics, Literature, and Informatics*. Chicago: U of Chicago P, 1999. Print.

Heath, Shirley Brice. *Ways with Words: Language, Life, and Work in Communities and Classrooms*. Cambridge: Cambridge UP, 1983. Print.

Hensley Owens, Kim. "Confronting Rhetorical Disability: A Critical Analysis of Women's Birth Plans." *Written Communication* 26.3 (2009): 247–72. Print.

———. "Revelations and Representations: Birth Stories and Motherhood on the Internet." *Textual Mothers/Maternal Texts: Motherhood in Contemporary Women's Literatures*. Ed. Elizabeth Podnieks and Andrea O'Reilly. West Waterloo, ON: Wilfred Laurier UP, 2009. 349–64. Print.

———. "Reviews and Reactions: A Rhetorical-Cultural Analysis of *The Business of Being Born*." *Rhetoric Review* 30.3 (2011): 293–311. Print.

———. "Rhetorics of E-Health and Information Age Medicine: A Risk-Benefit Analysis." *JAC* 31.1–2 (2011): 225–35. Print.

Hess, David J. *Science Studies: An Advanced Introduction*. New York: New York UP, 1997. Print.

Hodder, Ian. "The Interpretation of Documents and Material Culture." *Handbook of Qualitative Research*. Ed. Norman K. Denzin and Yvonna S. Lincoln. Thousand Oaks, CA: Sage, 2000. 703–16. Print.

Honig, Alice S., Hiram E. Fitzgerald, and Holly Brophy-Herb, eds. *Infancy in America: An Encyclopedia*. Vol. 1, *A–I*. ABC CLIO. *Googlebooks*. 2001. Web. 18 May 2011.

Hosseini, Khaled. *The Kite Runner*. New York: Riverhead, 2003. Print.

Hoyert, Donna L., Melonie Heron, Sherry L. Murphy, and Hsiang-Ching Kung. "Deaths: Final Data for 2003." *NCHA Health E-Stat*. Centers for Disease Control and Prevention. 7 Jan. 2010. Web. 2 Feb. 2012.

Huff, Cynthia A. "Textual Boundaries: Space in Nineteenth-Century Women's Manuscript Diaries." *Inscribing the Daily: Critical Essays on Women's Diaries*. Ed. Suzanne L. Bunkers and Cynthia A. Huff. Amherst: U of Massachusetts P, 1996. 123–38. Print.

Iovine, Vicki. *The Girlfriends' Guide to Pregnancy*. New York: Pocket Books, 1995. Print.

James, Henry. *Washington Square*. New York: Harper and Brothers, 1901. Print.

Jennifer. "Mary Cassandra Eliana." *TheLaborofLove.com*. n.d. Web. 5 Dec. 2005.

Jenny. "Zachary's Birth Story." *TheLaborofLove.com*. n.d. Web. 30 Nov. 2005.

Jess. "A Baby and Promotion All in One Day." *BirthStories.com*. n.d. Web. 5 Dec. 2005.

Jesse. "Birth Story of Jenna." *Plomp.com*. 16 Dec. 2004. Web. 30 Nov. 2005.

Johnson, Kenneth C., and Betty-Anne Daviss. "Outcomes of Planned Home Births with Certified Professional Midwives: Large Prospective Study in North America." *British Medical Journal* 330 (2005): 1416–23. Print.

Jones, Terry, dir. *Monty Python's The Meaning of Life*. MCA, 1991. Film.

Jordan, Brigitte. *Birth in Four Cultures: A Crosscultural Investigation of Childbirth in Yucatan, Holland, Sweden, and the United States*. 3rd ed. Montreal: Eden Press, 1983. Print.

———. "Technology and the Social Distribution of Knowledge: Issues for Primary Health Care in Developing Countries." *Anthropology and Primary Health Care*. Ed. Jeannine Coreil and J. Dennis Mull. Boulder: Westview, 1990. 98–120. Print.

Joseph's mother. "Joseph's Birth." *Childbirth.org*. n.d. Web. 6 Dec. 2005.

Julie. "Birth Story of Devin Christopher." *Plomp.com*. 6 Jan. 2002. Web. 6 Dec. 2005.

Karen. "James David's Arrival." *UnassistedChildbirth.com*. n.d. Web. 5 Dec. 2005.

Keränen, Lisa. "'Cause Someday We All Die': Rhetoric, Agency, and the Case of the 'Patient' Preferences Worksheet." *Quarterly Journal of Speech* 93.2 (2007): 179–210. Web. 21 June 2011.

Kim. "Birth Story of Joshua Bradley Doering." *Plomp.com*. n.d. Web. 26 Jan. 2006.

Kirsch, Gesa. "Methodological Pluralism." *Methods and Methodology in Composition Research*. Ed. Gesa Kirsch and Patricia Sullivan. Carbondale: Southern Illinois UP, 1992. 247–69. Print.

Kirsch, Gesa and Patricia Sullivan, eds. *Methods and Methodology in Composition Research*. Carbondale: Southern Illinois UP, 1992. Print.

Kitzinger, Sheila. *Birth Crisis*. New York: Routledge, 2006. Print.

Klaus, Marshall H., and John H. Kennell. *Maternal-Infant Bonding*. St. Louis: C. V. Mosby, 1976. Print.

Klineman, Arthur, MD. *The Illness Narratives: Suffering, Healing, and the Human Condition*. New York: Basic, 1988. Print.

Koerber, Amy. "Postmodernism, Resistance, and Cyberspace: Making Rhetorical Spaces for Feminist Mothers on the Web." *Women's Studies* 24.2 (2001): 218–40. Print.

———. "Rhetorical Agency, Resistance, and the Disciplinary Rhetorics of Breastfeeding." *Technical Communication Quarterly* 15.1 (2006): 87–101. Print.

Kopelson, Karen. "Writing Patients' Wrongs: The Rhetoric and Reality of Information Age Medicine." *JAC* 29.1–2 (2009): 353–404. Print.

Krystle. "First Baby, Epidural, Easy." *BirthStories.com*. n.d. Web. 27 Jan. 2006.

Kuhn, Thomas. *The Structure of Scientific Revolutions*. 1962. Chicago: U of Chicago P, 1969. Print.

Kym. "Home Sweet Home Home." *UnasssistedChildbirth.com*. 1997. Web. 18 Dec. 2005.

Lang, Raven. *Birth Book*. Palo Alto, CA: Genesis, 1972. Print.

Lanham, Richard A. *The Electronic Word: Democracy, Technology, and the Arts.* Chicago: U of Chicago P, 1993. Print.

Laura Joy. "Zachary—Having a Baby 'on the Way!'" *UnassistedChildbirth.com.* n.d. Web. 30 Nov. 2005.

Laurie. "Angelica's Birth Story." *Childbirth.org.* 1997. Web. 6 Oct. 2005.

———. "An Ordinary Miracle." *UnassistedChildbirth.com.* n.d. Web. 14 Jan. 2011.

Lay, Mary M. "Midwives' Birth Stories: Narratives That Expand the Borders of Professional Discourse." *Narrative and Professional Communication.* Ed. Nancy Blyler and Jane Perkins. Stamford, CT: Ablex, 1999. 137–50. Print.

———. *The Rhetoric of Midwifery: Gender, Knowledge, and Power.* New Brunswick, NJ: Rutgers UP, 2000. Print.

Layne, Linda L. *Motherhood Lost: A Feminist Account of Pregnancy Loss in America.* New York: Routledge, 2003. Print.

Leavitt, Judith Walzer. *Brought to Bed: Childbearing in America, 1750 to 1950.* New York: Oxford UP, 1986. Print.

———. *Make Room for Daddy: The Journey from Waiting Room to Birthing Room.* Chapel Hill: U of North Carolina P, 2009. Print.

Lessl, Thomas M. "The Culture of Science and the Rhetoric of Scientism: From Francis Bacon to the Darwin Fish." *Quarterly Journal of Speech* 93.2 (2007): 123–49. Print.

Litoff, Judy Barrett. *American Midwives: 1860 to the Present.* Westport, CT: Greenwood, 1978. Print.

Liu, Yameng. "Invention and Inventiveness: A Postmodern Redaction." *Perspectives on Rhetorical Invention.* Ed. Janet M. Atwill and Janice M. Lauer. Knoxville: U of Tennessee P, 2002. 53–63. Print.

Loudon, Irvine. *Death in Childbirth: An International Study of Maternal Care and Maternal Mortality, 1800–1950.* Oxford: Clarendon Press, 1992. Print.

Lucas, George, dir. and writer. *Star Wars: Revenge of the Sith.* 2005. Lucasfilm and Twentieth Century Fox. Film.

Martin, Emily. *The Woman in the Body.* Boston: Beacon, 1987. Print.

Martin, George R. R. *A Game of Thrones.* New York: Bantam, 1997. Print.

Martin, Joyce A., et al. "Births: Final Data for 2004." *National Vital Statistics Reports, Centers for Disease Control and Prevention* 55.1 (2004). 1–102. Web. 19 July 2011.

———. "Births: Final Data for 2006." *National Vital Statistics Reports, Centers for Disease Control and Prevention* 57.7 (2006): 1–102. Web. 2 Feb. 2008.

Martin, Luther H., Huck Gutman, and Patrick H. Hutton, eds. *Technologies of the Self: A Seminar with Michel Foucault.* Amherst: U of Massachusetts P, 1988. Print.

McAdams, Dan. *Power, Intimacy, and the Life Story: Personological Inquiries into Identity.* New York: Guilford, 1988. Print.

Melissa. "Laurel's Birth Story." *TheLaborofLove.com.* 11 Feb. 2009 (n.d. when originally retrieved in 2005). Web. 5 Feb. 2012.

Mentor, Steven. "IVF, ART, and Complex Agency in the World of Techno Birth." *Cyborg Babies: From Techno-Sex to Techno-Tots.* Ed. Robbie Davis-Floyd and Joseph Dumit. New York: Routledge, 1998. 67–89. Print.

Meyer, Michaela. "Women Speak(ing): Forty Years of Feminist Contributions to Rhetoric and an Agenda for Feminist Rhetorical Studies." *Communication Quarterly* 55.1 (2007): 1–17. Web. 23 Mar. 2011.

Michel, Jean-Baptiste, et al. "Culturomics." *Culturomics.org.* 2010. Web. 18 May 2010.

———. "Quantitative Analysis of Culture Using Millions of Digitized Books." *Science* 331 (2011): 176–82. Web. 15 May 2010.

Mintz, Steven. "Childbirth in Early America." *Digital History.* 7 Feb. 2012. Web. 7 Feb. 2012.

Mitchell, Lisa M., and Eugenia Georges. "Baby's First Picture: The Cyborg Fetus of Ultrasound Imaging." *Cyborg Babies: From Techno Sex to Techno Tots.* Ed. Robbie Davis-Floyd and Joseph Dumit. New York: Routledge, 1998. 105–24. Print.

Mitford, Jessica. *The American Way of Birth.* New York: Dutton, 1992. Print.

Mizuno, K., N. Mizuno, T. Shinohara, and M. Noda. "Mother-Infant Skin-to-Skin Contact after Delivery Results in Early Recognition of Own Mother's Milk Odour." *Acta Pædiatrica* 93.12 (2004): 1560–62. Web. PubMed. 15841774.

Moraga, Cherrie. *Waiting in the Wings: Portrait of a Queer Motherhood.* Ithaca: Firebrand, 1997. Print.

Morris, T., and K. McInerney. "Media Representations of Pregnancy and Childbirth: An Analysis of Reality Television Programs in the United States." *Birth* 37.2 (2010): 134–40. Print.

National Society of Daughters of the American Revolution. *Daughters of the American Revolution Magazine* 81 (1947): 102. *Googlebooks.* Web. 18 May 2011.

Neisser, Ulrich. "Self-Narratives: True and False." *The Remembering Self: Construction and Accuracy in the Self-Narrative.* Ed. Ulrich Neisser and Robyn Fivush. Cambridge: Cambridge UP, 1994. 1–18. Print.

Newkirk, Thomas. "Seduction and Betrayal in Qualitative Research." *Ethics and Representation in Qualitative Studies of Literacy.* Ed. Gesa E. Kirsch and Peter Mortensen. Urbana: NCTE, 1996. 3–16. Print.

Nystrand, Martin, and John Duffy, eds. *Towards a Rhetoric of Everyday Life: New Directions in Research on Writing, Text, and Discourse.* Madison: U of Wisconsin P, 2003. Print.

Oakley, Ann. *Women Confined: Toward a Sociology of Childbirth.* New York: Schocken, 1980. Print.

"An OB's Birth Plan." *AllNurses.com.* 4 May 2009. Web. 30 Sept. 2011.

"Online Birth Planner." *Birthplan.com.* n.d. Web. 5 May 2006.

Osterman, Michelle J. K., and Joyce A. Martin. "Epidural and Spinal Anesthesia Use during Labor: 27-State Reporting Area, 2008." *National Vital Statistics Reports* 59.5 (2011): 3. Web. 30 Jan. 2012.

"Our Birth Plan." *Mjbovo.com.* n.d. Web. 15 Apr. 2005.

Paget, Marianne, and Marjorie L. DeVault. *A Complex Sorrow: Reflections on Cancer and an Abbreviated Life.* Philadelphia: Temple UP, 1993. Print.

Pennebaker, James W. *Opening Up: The Healing Power of Confiding in Others.* New York: Avon, 1990. Print.

Pitt, Susan. *Midwifery and Medicine: Gendered Knowledge in the Practice of Delivery.* London: Routledge, 1997. Print.

Plomp, Karen. "Birth Stories!!!" *Plomp.com.* 4 Apr. 2005. Web. 17 Nov. 2005.

———. "Birth Story of Tamara." *Plomp.com.* Web. 5 Dec. 2005.

Pollock, Della. *Telling Bodies Performing Birth: Everyday Narratives of Childbirth.* New York: Columbia UP, 1999. Print.

"Post Your Story on BirthStories.Com!" *BirthStories.com.* 2004. Web. 31 Oct. 2004.

Prendergast, Catherine. "On the Rhetorics of Mental Disability." *Towards a Rhetoric of Everyday Life: New Directions in Research on Writing, Text, and Discourse.* Ed. Martin Nystrand and John Duffy. Madison: U of Wisconsin P, 2003. 189–206. Print.

———. "Race: The Absent Presence in Composition Studies." *College Composition and Communication* 50.1 (1998): 36–53. JSTOR. Web. 10 Mar. 2012.

"Privacy Policy Statement." *iParenting.com.* n.d. Web. 13 Dec. 2005.

"Purpose of a Birth Plan." *LSU Law Center's Medical and Public Health Law Site.* n.d. Web. 20 Nov. 2004.

Rachael. "Birth Story of Sammi." *Plomp.com.* 10 July 2001. Web. 20 Nov. 2005.

Rapp, Rayna. *Testing Women, Testing the Fetus: The Social Impact of Amniocentesis in America.* New York: Routledge, 1999. Print.

Ratcliffe, Krista. "Bearing Witness to Birth: A Literary Perspective." *Who's Having This Baby? Perspectives on Birthing.* Ed. Carla H. Hay, Helen M. Sterk, Alice. B. Kehoe, Krista Ratcliffe, and Leona G. Vandevusse. East Lansing: Michigan State UP, 2002. 43–86. Print.

———. "In Search of the Unstated: The Enthymeme and/of Whiteness." *JAC* 27.1 (2007): 275–89. Print.

Reagan, Leslie J. "From Hazard to Blessing to Tragedy: Representations of Miscarriage in Twentieth-Century America." *Feminist Studies* 29.2 (2003): 357–76. Print.

Rich, Adrienne Cecile. *Of Woman Born: Motherhood as Experience and Institution*. New York: Norton, 1976. Print.

Rooks, Judith Pence. *Midwifery and Childbirth in America*. Philadelphia: Temple UP, 1997. Print.

Ross, Michael, and Roger Buehler. "Creative Remembering." *The Remembering Self: Construction and Accuracy in the Self-Narrative*. Ed. Ulrich Neisser and Robyn Fivush. Cambridge: Cambridge UP, 1994. 205–35. Print.

Roth, Bobby, dir. "The Man behind the Curtain." *Lost*, 9 May 2007. Television.

Rowling, J. K. *Harry Potter and the Philosopher's Stone*. London: Bloomsbury Publishing, 1997. Print.

Sandra. "Birth Story of Colin." *Plomp.com*. 1 Jan. 2002. Web. 5 Mar. 2005.

Sandy. "Zachary Kyle Lee Thomson." *Childbirth.org*. 1999. Web. 2 Dec. 2005.

Santos, Marc C. "How the Internet Saved My Daughter and How Social Media Saved My Family." *Kairos* 15.2 (2011): n.pj. Web. 23 Feb. 2011.

Scarry, Elaine. *The Body in Pain: The Making and Unmaking of the World*. Cambridge: Oxford UP, 1987. Print.

Schuster, Mary Lay. "A Different Place to Birth: A Material Rhetoric Analysis of Baby Haven, a Free-Standing Birth Center." *Women's Studies in Communication* 29.1 (2006): 1–19. Print.

Scott, Amy. "Eyes-Open Childbirth: Writing a Meaningful Plan for a Gentle Birth." *TheLaborofLove.com*. n.d. Web. 30 May 2007.

Scott, J. Blake. *Risky Rhetoric: AIDS and the Cultural Practices of HIV Testing*. Carbondale: Southern Illinois UP, 2003. Print.

Scott, Joan W. "The Evidence of Experience." *Critical Inquiry* 17 (1991): 773–97. Print.

Scott, Kathryn D., Phyllis H. Klaus, and Marshall H. Klaus. "The Obstetrical and Postpartum Benefits of Continuous Support during Childbirth." *Journal of Women's Health and Gender-Based Medicine* 8.10 (1999): 1257–64. Print.

Sears, William, and Martha Sears. *The Birth Book: Everything You Need to Know to Have a Safe and Satisfying Birth*. Boston: Little, Brown, 1994. Print.

Segal, Judy Z. *Health and the Rhetoric of Medicine*. Carbondale: Southern Illinois UP, 2005. Print.

———. "Internet Health and the 21st-Century Patient." *Written Communication* 26.4 (2009): 351–69. Print.

Seigel, Marika. *Reproductive Technologies: Pregnancy Manuals as Technical Communication*. Diss. Pennsylvania State University, 2006. Print.

———. *The Rhetoric of Pregnancy*. Chicago: U of Chicago P, 2013. Print.

Shaw, Rhonda. "The Ethics of the Birth Plan in Childbirth Management Practices." *Feminist Theory* 3.2 (2002): 131–49. Print.

Shelley, Mary Wollstonecraft. *Frankenstein*. 1818. West Haven, CT: Pendulum Press, 1973. Print.

Sherry. "Mariah Elizabeth Kennedy's Birth." *Childbirth.org*. n.d. Web. 30 Nov. 2006.

Sherry. "Our Birth Story." *Plomp.com*. 27 Mar. 2001. Web. 5 Mar. 2005.

Sinor, Jennifer. *The Extraordinary Work of Ordinary Writing*. Iowa City: U of Iowa P, 2002. Print.

Smith, John E. "Time and Qualitative Time." *Rhetoric and* Kairos*: Essays in History, Theory, and Praxis*. Ed. Philip Sipiora and James E. Baumlin. Albany: SUNY P, 2002. 46–57. Print.

Spoel, Philippa. "Communicating Values, Valuing Community through Health-Care Websites: Midwifery's Online Ethos and Public Communication in Ontario." *Technical Communication Quarterly* 17.3 (2008): 264–88. Print.

———. "How Do Midwives Talk with Women? The Rhetorical Genre of Informed Choice in Midwifery." *Rhetorical Questions in Health and Medicine*. Ed. J. Leach and D. Dysart-Gale. New York: Rowman and Littlefield, 2010. 97–128. Print.

Stabile, Carol. "Shooting the Mother: Fetal Photography and the Politics of Disappearance." *The Visible Woman: Imaging Technologies, Gender, and Science*. Ed. Lisa Cartwright, Paula A. Treichler, and Constance Penley. New York: New York UP, 1998. 171–97. Print.

Stacy. "Peaceful Surrender." *Bornfree.com*. n.d. Web. 15 Oct. 2005.

Sullivan, Patricia, and James E. Porter. *Opening Spaces: Writing Technologies and Critical Research Practices*. Greenwich, CT: Ablex, 1997. Print.

Summer. "An Amazing Drug-Free Hypnobirth." *BirthStories.com*. n.d. Web. 5 Dec. 2006.

Susan. "Birth of My Gina." *TheLaborofLove.com*. n.d. Web. 18 Dec. 2005.

Sydney's mother. "Birth Story of Sydney." *Plomp.com*. 7 Feb. 2002. Web. 15 Nov. 2006.

Tague, Robert G. "Maternal Mortality or Prolonged Growth: Age at Death and Pelvic Size in Three Prehistoric Amerindian Populations." *American Journal of Physical Anthropology* 95 (1994): 27–40. PubMed. Web. 14 Feb. 2007.

Taylor, Catherine. *Giving Birth: A Journey into the World of Mothers and Midwives*. New York: Penguin, 2002. Print.

Taylor, Janelle S., Linda L. Layne, and Danielle F. Wozniak. *Consuming Motherhood*. New Brunswick, NJ: Rutgers UP, 2004. Print.

"Terms of Use." *TheLaborofLove.com*. n.d. Web. 16 Nov. 2005.

Tharp, Julie, and Susan MacCallum-Whitcomb. *This Giving Birth*. Bowling Green, OH: Bowling Green State University Popular Press, 2000. Print.

Thomas's mother. "Thomas Hall's Birth." *Childbirth.org*. n.d. Web. 6 Feb. 2006.

Treichler, Paula A. "Feminism, Medicine, and the Meaning of Childbirth." *Body/Politics, Women and the Discourses of Science*. Ed. Mary Jacobus, Evelyn Fox Keller, and Sally Shuttleworth. New York: Routledge, 1990. 113–38. Print.

Tucker, Holly. *Pregnant Fictions: Childbirth and the Fairy Tale in Early-Modern France*. Detroit: Wayne State UP, 2003. Print.

Tulsky, James A. "Beyond Advance Directives: Importance of Communication Skills at the End of Life." *Journal of the American Medical Association* 294 (2005): 359–65. Print.

Ulrich, Laurel Thatcher. *A Midwife's Tale: The Life of Martha Ballard, Based on Her Diary, 1785–1812*. New York: Knopf, 1991. Print.

Wagner, Marsden. *Born in the USA: How a Broken Maternity System Must Be Fixed to Put Women and Children First*. Berkeley: U of California P, 2006. Print.

Watts, Richard J. *Politeness*. New York: Cambridge UP, 2003. Print.

Weerasekera, D. S. "The Role of Forceps in Modern Obstetrics." *Journal of Obstetrics and Gynecology* 19.2 (1999): 146–49. Print.

Weiss, Robin Elise. "A Birth Plan: What Is That?" *Pregnancy.about.com*. n.d. Web. 18 July 2005.

Wells, Susan. *Our Bodies, Ourselves and the Work of Writing*. Stanford: Stanford UP, 2010. Print.

Wertz, Richard W., and Dorothy C. Wertz. *Lying-In: A History of Childbirth in America*. New Haven: Yale UP, 1989. Print.

"WHOIS Behind That Domain?" *Network Solutions*. N.p. 2010. Web. 19 Nov. 2010.

Wilgoren, Jodi. "'Mothering the Mother' during Childbirth, and After." *New York Times. Nytimes.com*. 25 Sept. 2005. Web. 25 Sept. 2005.

Wolf, Naomi. *Misconceptions: Truth, Lies, and the Unexpected on the Journey to Motherhood*. New York: Doubleday, 2001. Print.

Zerubavel, Eviatar. *Patterns of Time in Hospital Life: A Sociological Perspective*. Chicago: U of Chicago P, 1979. Print.

———. *Time Maps: Collective Memory and the Social Shape of the Past*. Chicago: U of Chicago P, 2003. Print.

INDEX

Italicized page numbers indicate figures and tables.

KIM HENSLEY OWENS is the director of composition and an associate professor of English at Northern Arizona University. Her *Written Communication* article won the 2010 SAGE New Scholar Award. Recent publications include articles in *Computers and Composition*, *Rhetoric Review*, *Enculturation*, and *Pedagogy* and chapters in *Textual Mothers/Maternal Texts* and *Writing Majors*.

Studies in Rhetorics and Feminisms

Studies in Rhetorics and Feminisms seeks to address the interdisciplinarity that rhetorics and feminisms represent. Rhetorical and feminist scholars want to connect rhetorical inquiry with contemporary academic and social concerns, exploring rhetoric's relevance to current issues of opportunity and diversity. This interdisciplinarity has already begun to transform the rhetorical tradition as we have known it (upper-class, agonistic, public, and male) into regendered, inclusionary rhetorics (democratic, dialogic, collaborative, cultural, and private). Our intellectual advancements depend on such ongoing transformation.

Rhetoric, whether ancient, contemporary, or futuristic, always inscribes the relation of language and power at a particular moment, indicating who may speak, who may listen, and what can be said. The only way we can displace the traditional rhetoric of masculine-only, public performance is to replace it with rhetorics that are recognized as being better suited to our present needs. We must understand more fully the rhetorics of the non-Western tradition, of women, of a variety of cultural and ethnic groups. Therefore, Studies in Rhetorics and Feminisms espouses a theoretical position of openness and expansion, a place for rhetorics to grow and thrive in a symbiotic relationship with all that feminisms have to offer, particularly when these two fields intersect with philosophical, sociological, religious, psychological, pedagogical, and literary issues.

The series seeks scholarly works that both examine and extend rhetoric, works that span the sexes, disciplines, cultures, ethnicities, and sociocultural practices as they intersect with the rhetorical tradition. After all, the recent resurgence of rhetorical studies has been not so much a discovery of new rhetorics as a recognition of existing rhetorical activities and practices, of our newfound ability and willingness to listen to previously untold stories.

The series editors seek both high-quality traditional and cutting-edge scholarly work that extends the significant relationship between rhetoric and feminism within various genres, cultural contexts, historical periods, methodologies, theoretical positions, and methods of delivery (e.g., film and hypertext to elocution and preaching).

Queries and submissions:

Professor Cheryl Glenn, Editor
E-mail: cjg6@psu.edu
Professor Shirley Wilson Logan, Editor
E-mail: slogan@umd.edu

Studies in Rhetorics and Feminisms

Department of English
142 South Burrowes Bldg.
Penn State University
University Park, PA 16802-6200

Other Books in the Studies in Rhetorics and Feminisms Series

A Feminist Legacy: The Rhetoric and Pedagogy of Gertrude Buck
Suzanne Bordelon

Regendering Delivery: The Fifth Canon and Antebellum Women Rhetors
Lindal Buchanan

Rhetorics of Motherhood
Lindal Buchanan

Conversational Rhetoric: The Rise and Fall of a Women's Tradition, 1600–1900
Jane Donawerth

Feminism beyond Modernism
Elizabeth A. Flynn

Women and Rhetoric between the Wars
Edited by Ann George, M. Elizabeth Weiser, and Janet Zepernick

Educating the New Southern Woman: Speech, Writing, and Race at the Public Women's Colleges, 1884–1945
David Gold and Catherine L. Hobbs

Women's Irony: Rewriting Feminist Rhetorical Histories
Tarez Samra Graban

The Rhetoric of Rebel Women: Civil War Diaries and Confederate Persuasion
Kimberly Harrison

Evolutionary Rhetoric: Sex, Science, and Free Love in Nineteenth-Century Feminism
Wendy Hayden

Liberating Voices: Writing at the Bryn Mawr Summer School for Women Workers
Karyn L. Hollis

Gender and Rhetorical Space in American Life, 1866–1910
Nan Johnson

Appropriate[ing] Dress: Women's Rhetorical Style in Nineteenth-Century America
Carol Mattingly

The Gendered Pulpit: Preaching in American Protestant Spaces
Roxanne Mountford

Rhetorical Listening: Identification, Gender, Whiteness
Krista Ratcliffe

Feminist Rhetorical Practices: New Horizons for Rhetoric, Composition, and Literacy Studies
Jacqueline J. Royster and Gesa E. Kirsch

Vote and Voice: Women's Organizations and Political Literacy, 1915–1930
Wendy B. Sharer

Women Physicians and Professional Ethos in Nineteenth-Century America
Carolyn Skinner